Nightmares Can Come True

Inside the Head and Heart of Grief

Mrs. Dixon,

You have always been so supportive and always seem to have a smile on your face. It's people like you that make HSES such an amazing place to work and that was so huge in my survival. Thanks for being you.

—Levi 10-30-20

Nightmares Can Come True

Inside the Head and Heart of Grief

Levi Moore

Levi Moore

ISBN: 978-1-944662-52-3

Publishing date: September 2020

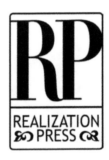

Cover Design by Othman Attaf

Dedication

This book is dedicated to Denise Halsey Moore.

Contents

Chapter 1
Our Love

Denise and my life will always be a love story followed by tragedy. Many people experience the type of story that mirrors the first four years we were together. Few know the amount of happiness and pure joy we shared in our last year together. Hardly anyone goes through the kind of ending we had.

2011 – 2015

Denise and I first met teaching together at the same school. Denise was a resident of Raleigh, North Carolina, and I had just moved into town after working on my master's degree at East Carolina University. We had seen each other at school and in trainings but were so focused on the new set of students we had we didn't start talking until a couple months into school.

After those couple of months, some of our co-workers would get together after school hours, and I immediately felt attracted to Denise. I already had seen how wonderful she was with her students, and her smile was really something beautiful. During an evening of watching a co-worker's band play, I learned that she too was single. I talked with her, and the next evening I asked her out. Luckily she agreed to be seen with me in public.

Our first date was to dinner and to see the movie *Tower Heist*. We had a really good time and laughed a good amount together. Very soon after our successful first date, she agreed to let me take her out for a second. For that date we shared dinner again and then made a trip to a library to get me a biography we had talked about during one of our book discussions.

Since I was 29 and Denise was 34, we both were looking for a longer relationship and found happiness with each other. We started to hang out together on weekends, and soon I spent many of my Saturday evenings at her apartment, eating Papa Murphy's take-and-bake pizza and playing cards. We learned early on that we were both looking for someone with whom to build a life. After only a few months of dating, knowing that we were both deeply in love, we purchased a house in south Raleigh.

We moved about 10 minutes away from Denise's sister, Dawn, brother-in-law Brian, and niece Sara. Our home was wonderful and we loved being so near her sister and her family. Within a couple more months, her parents, Bill and Judy, decided they too wanted to be closer to their two daughters and built a house in the same development as ours. Denise and I spent many Saturday nights at her parents' eating dinner, playing the card game Euchre, and laughing well into the evening.

A proposal soon followed and a wedding date was set. At the wedding, Denise looked beautiful. She always had a great smile but on that day between the sun, her brown hair falling down to her beautiful white dress, and that smile, she was really the most beautiful bride. She had waited a long time to be the bride and really seemed to enjoy the moment. At the wedding everyone had a great time and we were incredible lucky with such a perfect day. A highlight of the wedding was one of my special education students, Davis, welcoming all the guests from his wheelchair and passing out bulletins to our wonderful family and friends.

Denise and I honeymooned in Cancun, Mexico. We loved being together and enjoyed the breathtaking scenery. Every moment we built memories.

We were overjoyed by how quickly our lives merged and how comfortable we felt being a couple. We did almost everything together. Every Friday after school we went grocery shopping. We played many games together and our favorite tradition became our yearly winter break card and board game tournament, which ended with bowling on New Year's Day.

Denise and I had built an amazing life in a brief amount of time. We loved being alone together, but we also treasured spending time with her family. We spent many vacations with her family, and, on almost all of them, we stayed with Dawn, Brian, and Sara or with Bill and Judy.

Denise and I were deeply in love and profoundly happy. However, there was one thing that was missing in our lives, and this was a huge void in Denise's heart. For quite a while, we had been trying to have a child. Denise found it difficult to see so many of her younger friends become pregnant while she remained childless. This was challenging for both of us, and it was the only thing missing from our lives. In my heart,

I knew that Denise and I both loved each other and that we could be okay without kids. However, I always assumed that we would end up with children of our own whom we would love and cherish.

2016

This year marks one of the happiest and saddest times of my life. This was the last year I was with Denise, but, up until her death, it was everything we could have hoped for and more.

Denise and I continued to struggle both emotionally and financially with our attempts to have children. We had spent a good amount of time talking about our future, and the thought of sharing a life without children had crept into our minds. We both hoped this would not be the case but recognized there was a chance that our life together might be empty.

We had lived in our house for about four years and really enjoyed it. It was our home and it was beautiful. However, the property had a couple of issues. First, we didn't have much of a backyard, and we always envisioned having an area for our kid(s) to play. Secondly, our house backed up to the main entrance of the neighborhood, and often neighbors would wake us with speeding cars, and we found it difficult to get back to sleep. Other than these two challenges, we could have stayed in that house forever.

Denise had gotten the idea of trying to sell the house and buy a new one in our neighborhood closer to the back of the subdivision. Honestly, I didn't know if we could get the price we wanted and knew that our finances were not what I liked for such a big undertaking. I have to give Denise credit though;

when she put her mind to something, she was completely committed. Our friend Gus was in real estate and we asked him about trying to sell our house. He was interested and so began the process of putting our property on the market.

Our house had been for sale for some time, and, with the exception of a single, low-ball offer, there weren't many takers. As this was going on, we were looking at houses in the back of our subdivision. We really liked the neighborhood and thought this would be a great place to raise our children (if we were so lucky).

On February 1st we signed the papers to build our new home. It was an exciting time for Denise, but I remained a little worried about whether or not our house would sell. When we spoke to the building manager, she acted like she could save the house for a little while in case our house wouldn't sell. We felt it was definitely worth a shot and just hoped that someone would like our house enough to buy it within our price range. We would need the money from our old house to make the down payment on our new house. It was a little bit of a gamble, but it was worth the risk; plus to see Denise's smile was indeed priceless (corny, I know).

We celebrated Valentine's Day by cooking dinner and watching a movie. This was how we spent many weekends, but we still enjoyed our time being low-key and together. We even got to celebrate Denise's father's birthday the same weekend. All of this love that we shared as a whole family and between Denise and me was building up to our latest attempt at becoming parents. We had another doctor's appointment in early March and hoped this visit would turn out better than the previous ones.

The morning we were to receive Denise's pregnancy results, she went to the doctor's office and I headed to school.

I had agreed to take a half day off in hopes that we would get to celebrate with good news that afternoon. We had done this same routine a number of times before and each had ended in disappointment. We sincerely hoped that day would be different.

I got home and looked at Denise and she just looked at me. She told me to check my email and, sure enough, in my email was a forwarded message from Denise that concluded that we were pregnant. It was amazing! We were so grateful that the journey we had been on for so long was going to end in pure happiness. It was an amazing feeling. It was an unforgettable moment. To celebrate, Denise had already purchased a book for me about being a father. It was one of those rare moments in life that seems to be pure bliss.

As excited as we were, I was afraid her mom was going to have a heart attack. Judy could get emotional to say the least. This was something that might explode her heart. We walked to her parents' house and shared the good news. There were tears and smiles and everything seemed to be falling into place. Denise and I were incredibly lucky. I reminded us both that, as good as our story was turning out, there were many people who never got the news we received that day, and because of that we should be even more thankful for what we had. It was a day beyond description.

Later in March we had plans to spend a week in Orlando with her parents. Bill and Judy had a timeshare and they agreed to let us come with them. This trip was planned well before our good news, and it was set up as either an escape after finding out once again we weren't pregnant or a celebration of being pregnant. Luckily for us, the trip was for the second reason. We just hung out at the resort and played a lot of cards. We went on some small trips around Orlando. Bill and I went to a golf tournament, which was part of his birthday present, and another day Denise and I took a trip to a retirement community called The Villages to see a former retired colleague of mine. It was a successful vacation apart from the loud kids on spring break that limited our sleep. Overall, we had a great time being together and celebrating Denise's pregnancy.

Things were definitely working out well for Denise and me. We still had the obstacle of trying to sell our house, but we were ecstatic with how things were going and then we got some even better news. After returning home from Orlando, Denise and I went in for a visit to the doctor and were given a huge shock. Not only would Denise be carrying one baby, she would be carrying two. Twins!

I will never forget sitting in that chair next to Denise when they said that she had two babies. This massive, dumb, goofy grin spread across my face. I seriously knew that if anyone saw my expression they would have thought I was a big idiot. I sat there gushing with excitement, and Denise was even more ecstatic. We left the doctor's office and called our parents, and there was happiness aplenty.

Denise and I spent the next couple of weeks discussing what we hoped the sexes of our kids would be. We agreed that as long as they were healthy we would be blessed. We felt the best-case scenario would be one boy and one girl. At that moment we couldn't have been happier with life. The year 2016 was turning out to be the most amazing one for us. Hopefully it would be the start of something special and amazing.

A couple weeks later we celebrated my birthday and, as was her way, Denise spent way too much money on me. After that we got more good news. We were sitting at breakfast when I received a text from our realtor Gus. He mentioned that he received an offer on our house. It was still lower than our asking price by quite a bit. We had been down this road before and knew that if we countered and there was a middle ground, we would be good. If we came back with a reasonable price but the buyer failed to meet us in the middle, then we probably wouldn't be selling the house to that individual.

After our counter, it was clear that we were going to be able to come to an agreement. We had cleared our next obstacle and sold the house. It was really the last step in our journey, and we just hoped everything else would work itself out. We continued to celebrate this move forward and hoped to welcome our children into this world with everything we had and held dearest.

Selling a house sounds great on paper. Once you realize that you have to clean everything, put all your belongings into boxes and actually move, you realize how exhausting it is. We were lucky to have her parents help us. During Memorial Day weekend, we spent a great deal of time trying to clean the entire place and put most of our belongings into boxes. You never really realize how much stuff you have accumulated over a short amount of time until you try to package it. We got a great deal of work completed that weekend, and, with the help of a garage sale and a couple of Pack Rat portable storage units, we were able to clear out the house in time for the closing.

Denise and I were having a great year and were fortunate things were turning out so well. Trying to figure out where we were going to live for a couple months was no exception.

Denise's parents agreed to let us stay with them between the selling of our old house and the closing of our new one. I got along beautifully with her parents, so I wasn't concerned about living with them. Denise and I agreed that for every month we stayed with Bill and Judy, we would pay for all the groceries. We actually all had a really good time. We played cards on weekends and watched all kinds of movies. We even got to hang out with their cocker spaniel Olaf. Coming home to a meal we didn't need to prepare was an added bonus. Denise and I enjoyed our time with Bill and Judy but were anxious to get into our new home and have everything settled in anticipation of the arrivals of our babies.

With our lives seemingly coming together, we still had one big surprise waiting for us. We didn't have any idea about the sex of the babies. We agreed to get one of those gender reveal cakes on Father's Day. Without looking at the results, Judy got someone to bake the cake, which was decorated with two elephants on top, one boy and one girl with a question mark in between. We couldn't wait to cut into the cake and find out what sexes our babies were going to be. I let Denise make the first slice as she was much better around knives than I was. When we pulled out the first piece of cake, we saw blue and pink. It felt pretty amazing to know at last. We were so excited to have a boy and a girl. We couldn't have asked for anything better. As long as they were healthy, we only hoped that we could make them happy babies. It was a beautiful moment that we were fortunate to share with her parents, family, and our friends. I will admit I felt weird eating the cake, but it was such a fun experience that Denise and I were glad we got to do together.

Although Denise and I enjoyed and appreciated our time with Bill, Judy, and Olaf, we were enthusiastic about getting into our house and putting it together in time for the twins' arrival. On August 3rd we closed on our new home. It was a wonderful experience and we were excited to get started settling in.

We had planned on having the first of the Pack Rat portable storage units dropped off that Saturday so that we could get everything unloaded from that one as quickly as possible. Luckily that Saturday it did not rain. Unfortunately for Denise and her parents, I had to attend a CPR training at school that Saturday. I was going to miss all the fun. However, I pulled my weight when I arrived home, getting the very few things left, mainly furniture, out with the help of a local retired strongman that Bill knew. One Pack Rat was empty and plenty of boxes awaited unpacking in the house. If we didn't have Bill and Judy to help us, I think we would have been in some serious trouble as Denise was very pregnant by that time, and she couldn't lift anything much or bend down at all. Denise and I were thankful to have her parents help us as much as they did both that day and every day.

After the second Pack Rat was delivered and emptied, we could begin to lay out the rooms the way we wanted them. We were lucky that we could measure the rooms while the house was being built and figure out which of our furniture to keep and what to sell. From there we were able to know what would go in every room, so, after the first couple of weekends, it was a lot of unpacking boxes and putting things away. The transition of the house went seamlessly and it worked out well.

Denise and I had previously talked about our car situation. She drove a Ford Fusion and I had a Honda CR-V. I told her all along that I wouldn't mind owning and driving a minivan, as my dad had one while I was a child and we took it on a number of trips. Denise was adamant that we would not be owning a minivan. Bummer. We decided on looking at a new Ford Explorer. We had previously spent a good amount of time looking at buying a new vehicle but couldn't do anything until our new house closed for the sake of our credit. We had set up an appointment after the closing.

That Saturday, we ate some dinner and went to look at cars. We didn't find exactly the vehicle we wanted. Denise was so good at being prepared, so we knew all our options and had a definite idea about what we hoped to buy. The salesman, who was the boyfriend of the girl we originally agreed to buy our car from, was wonderful and brought us up a new Ford Explorer. We knew buying a new one was going to be a little bit more money than a previous year's model, but, with my trade-in, if they could offer something around our price, it was a possibility. Sure enough we found a middle ground and agreed to purchase the vehicle. We were so excited about our new car that we forgot to remove the garage door opener from the CR-V. It all worked out and we had the vehicle that we would happily bring the children home from the hospital in.

With the new house and car, there really seemed to be only one last big step to get ready for our twins. Denise had dreamed of how to set up the nursery, and we were excited to piece it together. Soon after the closing of the house and the purchasing of the new car, our two cribs were delivered. We had the color schemes chosen and spent an evening building the cribs together. Denise wanted to help even though it was difficult for her to get down on the floor. She loved helping assemble the baby's new little beds. It was an enjoyable evening for the two of us, and, even though neither of us were particularly handy, the cribs turned out great, and we were excited to use them as soon as the little ones arrived.

Denise had looked forward to Labor Day weekend for a long time. Her sister, Dawn, had agreed to open her house and host the family and friends for Denise's baby shower. Both of our schools had generously given us each a shower, and they both were wonderful occasions. However, this was the big shower and Denise could not have been prouder to be the star attraction for the afternoon. A couple of us guys went downstairs and played some Nintendo games while she opened a lot of wonderful presents that would soon be used.

Denise and I seemed to get pretty much everything we needed. We found it joyful to discover how many of the presents were for the boy and how many were for the girl. Denise had attended so many baby showers in the past. Now it was great to see this be her day. She loved every minute of it and enjoyed all the wonderful presents. We both felt spoiled and looked forward to the time we would get to use all those gifts.

October 22nd was the last day I was able to spend with Denise. She had been out of school for a little over a month between her track out break and her maternity leave. We had everything ready to go. The car was packed, everything was laid out, the nursery was set up, and the last thing would be to go to the hospital. Sadly that experience never came.

I remember spending the day trying to take care of all the housework while Denise rested; this was our normal weekend routine. I was sitting down in the evening watching a Saturday football game with Denise by my side, looking down at her phone, when she started tearing up. I asked her what was wrong, and she told me she had passed her National Board Certification, a five-year certificate similar to a master's degree. Denise had agreed to try to re-up her current certificate and did so before we found out she was pregnant. Denise tried hard to complete the huge amount of work required during her first trimester.

I could see the jubilation in her eyes. I asked when she was supposed to find out whether or not she had passed. She said she didn't think she would get the news until close to Thanksgiving. She was thrilled to receive it so early.

I felt so proud of her. But I knew she should be relaxing, so I told her to stop checking her work email and just rest. It was a wonderful, clear memory. She called her parents to let them know the good news, and we ended up going over to see them and were joined by Dawn and Sara. We took joy in celebrating her accomplishment together.

At this point, Denise was only about 10 days away from her scheduled delivery date. However, she was so excited to be with her family, and, looking back on it, I could never have asked for a better way for her last meal. Denise felt uncomfortable but was happy to be with her family. We said our goodbyes at the end of the evening, and my beautiful wife and I came home to see what she hoped wasn't the last happy memory of the night.

Denise's family is from Chicago. They are big Cubs baseball fans. That night if the Cubs won, they would go to the World Series. The games were always on late, and Denise had planned to stay up and watch the game. I had been sleeping downstairs because her sleep was so scarce. I did my best not to wake her up when my morning alarm went off. However, before going downstairs, I lay next to her and watched a couple innings. Before leaving to go to bed, I kissed her goodnight and told her I would see her in the morning. Sadly that was the last time that I ever saw Denise alive. She was always a wonderful, thoughtful, and caring person. Her death will never change that. But, sadly for us, her death changed everything about our lives.

Chapter 2

The First Day

The next morning I woke up oblivious to what my day had in store for me. I rose fairly early as I generally do and played around on my phone before I got out of bed. The highlight was seeing that well after I had fallen asleep Denise had posted on Facebook that the Cubs were going to the World Series. It was great to wake up to see that.

I usually waited a little bit before I went in to see Denise so that she could sleep as long as possible. By this time in her pregnancy, she was so uncomfortable that sleep was difficult, and I often waited to wake her before leaving for work. On weekends she would always text me to let me know she was awake, and I would rush in to see my beautiful wife.

This morning I got up and had breakfast and brushed my teeth, cut up my apples for the week, and made my sandwich for the next day. There really wasn't much else to do for the house, but we did have a couple of car bases that needed to go into the Ford Fusion that I figured I would go ahead and put in. I remember putting them in that morning up until the port-a-potty for the workers building the new house across the street got emptied. I did a good amount of work and was happy that with my chores were complete, and I would get to spend the rest of the day with Denise.

About the time a London football game was coming on, 9:30 a.m., I went in to check on her. As I slowly opened the door, I looked for Denise. However, I first noticed that she wasn't in the bed. I actually got excited because for a second, I thought she was in the bathroom, which would mean she was up. However, as soon as that thought came into my head, I saw a couple black marks on the bed. I quickly opened the door wider to find that Denise had fallen out of bed and was now leaned up with her head against the nightstand.

I instantly knew something was wrong and quickly went for my phone. I was so nervous that it took me two tries to dial 9-1-1. I told the dispatcher the situation and was in such shock about the unfolding events. I was mindful enough to go downstairs and unlock the door for the medical professionals. I knew once I went into that room I wasn't leaving.

I described what I was seeing to the dispatcher about how Denise was leaned up against the nightstand and that she was pregnant and we needed someone to get to the house immediately. I told him that I had already unlocked the door and that they could come directly upstairs to where I would be. I described how there were black marks on the bed and wall and explained that Denise's mouth and tongue seemed to be expanded. I confirmed my address and the dispatcher instantly told me that people were on the way and that help would be there shortly.

The dispatcher said I should put the phone on speaker and position it by her and that I was going to need to do CPR on Denise. I tried really hard to pull her off the nightstand but did so with great gentleness, trying not to hurt her. She was heavy and the side of her face that leaned against the nightstand was darker than the other side. Still in shock, I didn't fully understand what was happening and tried to inform the dispatcher to see if he could call Bill and Judy to let them know there was a situation.

When I managed to move her on the carpet, her left arm was positioned behind her back, and I couldn't get it in front of her. I told the dispatcher about this, and he informed me that I would need to move her arm. I tried in vain to reposition her arm. The dispatcher told me I needed to be rougher, and I responded that I didn't want to hurt her.

"Don't worry about that now," the dispatcher said firmly. "You need to try to get her on her side."

I was pushing with all my might, but I couldn't get both the top half and bottom half of her body into position. Finally, the dispatcher told me to go ahead and start pushing on her chest while she was on her back. I began to push down over her heart as hard as I could and counted out loud 1-2-3-4 so the dispatcher could hear me.

I was trying to stay as strong as I could and keep going, but after some time I started getting tired. The dispatcher was yelling at me to continue and reassured me that help would be there shortly. I was growing increasingly exhausted and kept trying to push on the count, speaking louder to keep up long enough before help could arrive and get Denise talking.

As I continued to press on Denise's chest, I heard the sound of vehicles outside and soon people entered the house. I directed them upstairs, and the two emergency men arrived and came into the bedroom, assessed the situation, and asked me to go to the other room. I left expecting them to continue to try to help Denise.

Very shortly after I exited our bedroom, more people arrived, and soon after that an older gentleman asked me to sit down. He gave me the worst news I think anyone could hear.

Already weakened by shock, I felt as if I were sinking. I couldn't wrap my head around everything. As he told me that Denise was no longer alive, I couldn't fully cope with what was happening. Somewhere inside I knew something catastrophic had happened, but I still couldn't imagine its life-altering effects. I understood I was still breathing, still functioning, but I couldn't come to grips with the scope of my situation. I was aware of the people who were there but didn't grasp the gravity of what they clearly understood and I was still trying to process.

When I managed to choke out the words, I wasn't sure if I were actually speaking. "What about the babies," I said.

The man's voice was kind and filled with sadness. "They are no longer living," he said.

There are a lot of really bad things in this world. In this moment I was living one. Denise and I had built a beautiful life together. We did things the way they were supposed to be done. Now it was all gone.

I had no idea what to do. I wouldn't wish that conversation on anyone. It was the worst news any person could get.

The nice gentleman asked me about telling family. I thought of Bill and Judy, of Dawn and her family. I ached inside.

"I haven't been able to get hold of her parents. They need to know," I said. A thought came to me. "Bill and Judy might be in church. Yes, that's probably where they are."

From there it was all just sadness.

I called Dawn and, as anyone would, she reeled from the news. She was able to get someone to watch Sara so she could come over to the house as soon as possible.

More medical people kept coming into the house, and then the police arrived to do what they needed to do. A really good police officer sat me down in the loft, put his hand on my shoulder, and informed me that he would be asking me some difficult questions.

I told him as best I could that I didn't care how uncomfortable the questions he was going to ask were. I would tell him anything and everything because my job was to get back into the bedroom with Denise as quickly as I could.

We walked through everything. To say that each of those cops treated me with compassion and the utmost respect would be selling them short. Those police officers were the best of the best. Even in the worst moment of my life, I could recognize professional and personal care. They had a job to do and I'm sure none of them wanted to be there under those circumstances, but they did what they had to with the utmost respect toward both my situation and me. I showed the officer Denise's Facebook post about the Cubs to help identify a timeline.

There was protocol they needed to follow, and I had to be monitored for obvious reasons. I didn't quite know what to do or how to act. What I expressed was that I wanted to get back into that room as quickly as possible and for as long as I could.

All the EMTs and police were compassionate. At a certain point, they asked me to go outside with the rest of her family, who had been made to wait there until someone was able to come to take pictures. The only thing I grabbed from the house was a box we hadn't unpacked that contained our photobooks, all of our memories. I walked out of the house as pathetic as anyone has ever been into the waiting arms of her family.

We hugged and cried together. I didn't say much. They took a folding chair out of my brother-in-law's truck and let me sit in it and look at our photo albums as I cried. It was a monumentally difficult situation.

I learned later that some of the officers chose to sit in their cars because they didn't really have the words for the situation. No pain I had ever felt compared to the agony of these moments. Hopefully it will be the worst moment of my life; I can't imagine anything worse.

We all stayed quiet for a long while. I was just waiting until I could get the okay to go back into the house and be by her for however long they would let me. When I was finally given the okay, I went back into the house, up the stairs, and into the bedroom.

I felt the most unbelievable, crushing sadness. The cops needed to leave one person in the room to monitor the scene, Denise, and me. I completely understood and was just grateful that they gave me the last opportunity to be with Denise in the home that we built.

I have no idea how long I was with her, but I poured my heart out to her in those moments. I sat in the corner and leaned against the chest of drawers, talking to the woman I loved whose body was now draped in a white sheet. I gave her my very best, and I talked to her as if she were the most beautiful person I ever met, which she was.

For all those people who think their occupations are hard, just imagine the job that cop had as he stood there in that room with me, hearing me pour my heart out to Denise. It helped to express my innermost feelings to her. I tried my hardest to give her everything I had in life and after her life was taken.

I quickly realized there likely would be only a couple more times I would get to be with her, and this was the first of those opportunities. I talked my heart out and cried so much. The sadness was unrelenting. At a certain point, I was told that I would have to leave.

I went back outside and agreed that I would stay until she was loaded into the van and taken away. My brother-in-law remained with me while the rest of the family went back to Denise's parent's house.

My own parents were not with us yet. I had called them earlier. My father has never been short of words; however, this time he was. He later told me that when he saw I was calling that early in the morning, he assumed it was to tell him that we had the babies or were at the hospital. Imagine that swing of emotion. We were so close to having everything. Dad wouldn't be the only person who had that reaction.

My mom and dad were able to get their dog boarded so they could head over as soon as I told them the news. I cannot even imagine that seven-hour car ride, knowing the tragic circumstances they were going to face when they arrived.

Brian, my brother-in-law, and I stood in silence with the family gone. A van pulled up and a stretcher was taken in. When it came back out carrying Denise's body, I thanked each of the people for taking good care of my beautiful wife. When they left, Brian and I walked to Denise's parents' home. I didn't talk much and when we got to their house, I sat in their screened-in back porch with my photo albums. And there I stayed.

There was nothing to say. I just looked at our pictures, our memories, and cried. It was the most horrible thing I ever experienced. I was living in the darkness. I stayed on the porch and sometimes went for walks around the neighborhood. I did this off and on throughout the afternoon.

I was cognizant enough to call a couple friends and tell them the horrific news. I couldn't imagine being on the other end of the phone hearing that. I hated being the person who brought that news, to drop this sorrow into their world. Still, I was the one who had to live it.

During the day, I called my principal, who lived in the same neighborhood with us. She had been one of the first people to learn of the tragedy. The ambulance had driven right passed her back door, and instantly she texted me to make sure Denise and I were okay. I believe I sent her the worst and saddest text message anyone has ever delivered. In fact, while the police were interviewing me, Mrs. Clark was outside my house. I never saw her but the police officers were nice enough to let me know that she was there.

When I called her, she was already in one of those school meetings that no one wants to be a part of. Since Denise was a teacher, there were some things that the county needed to do to support the students in her class as well as the other employees at her school. I was able to talk to her, my assistant principal, as well as Denise's principal, and tell them what I could.

They had begun the first part of a crisis plan to better serve the students and staff following this tragedy. I told them everything I could, and I know they were in a really bad position, trying to deal with the professional side of death, but I'm sure that hearing what happened to Denise from my own mouth was way worse.

Denise and my life should never have ended that way. Sadly, it was up to everyone else to pick up the pieces and try to better prepare her staff and students for what was about to come. This was a Sunday, so they were able to better deal with some things since school wasn't in session. They had plans for how to deal with this kind of experience, but, like a lot of things, they hoped they never would have to use them.

Her principal and my administration were consoling and comforting, and, as I signed off, they let me know if I needed anything they would be there for me. Both Denise and I were lucky to work for such great people.

At one point, I was in Denise's parents' house when the pastors came in. Denise and I had visited the church that her parents attended a couple of times. I believe her parents were at church when I discovered Denise. The pastors introduced themselves and agreed to say a prayer for the family. I wasn't having any of it and marched back out the back door to the porch at the word "prayer."

When things like this happen, you can about imagine my views on religion. I decided to ignore the prayers for support and continued looking at all Denise and I had left, our memories.

Pastor Gene came out and sat across from me. He didn't say anything and I didn't have any words for him. Then a weird thing happened that brought us closer. His phone did the "Na-Na-Na, Na-Na-Na," the ESPN noise. If not for that sound, I probably wouldn't have said a word to him. I asked what that was and he said it was his ESPN app telling him something.

We didn't start off talking about my current situation; we did some simple fantasy football discussion. I know that it was the last thing we should have been talking about, but I also realized that it was the distraction I needed from a world of pain that I was entering. We spoke a little about football, which was going on, and he gave me his condolences. After a little while, both he and Pastor Valerie left, and I went back to my photo albums and walks in the neighborhood.

The family was extremely sweet to me, but we all understood that there was nothing to be said. There were just tears to be shed and questions that may never be answered. I went back outside and found myself walking by our old house. We were great friends with our neighbors there, who, like us, were pretty young.

When I knocked, Dave answered the door with the widest grin on his face, anxious to hear about the new little babies. I felt so empty telling him something had happened. He knew right away it was terrible. I can only imagine the feelings he had as he walked back into the house, holding his child, and coming out the garage door to avoid letting the dog loose. I told him about Denise's passing and the loss of the babies. The emptiness in his eyes was disheartening. I have always been a person who likes to keep things positive and tries to be as upbeat as I can. At that moment it was clear it would be a while till I could smile. The conversation we had was excruciating. After I told him and we chatted for a few minutes, I realized I had nothing else to say. I hugged him and continued on my walk.

The life Denise and I built turned out to be about five beautiful years. Our world was shattered in what was essentially our prime. Denise so desperately wanted children, and I so badly wanted to see her with kids. It's a true shame how everything turned out.

I still had no idea what to say or do. When my parents arrived, we shared more tears and sadness. I am very much a mold of my father. I can only really think of a couple of times that he has been truly sad. This was the beginning of seeing a side of my father I never wanted to know. My parents were some of the most sincere, no gossip, kind-hearted people, and they had just walked into a minefield of sadness, and their only son was the star of one of the worst shows in the world.

At some point, we all probably tried to eat something but never could. The rest of the day became a blur after that. There were more tears than words, and the worst part was that it was all just the beginning.

Looking back on it, I couldn't believe how lucky I was. I know it sounds wrong but, if Denise and I hadn't lived so close to her family, I would have had to remain in the house where Denise passed away. Having Bill and Judy so close turned out to be the best blessing in the worst of times. At least we were all together, and, whatever the rest of the week had in store for us, we were going to cross that barrier together.

As the evening wore on, we all felt exhausted. It was simply the worst day of all of our lives and we lived it together. My parents and I stayed with Bill and Judy that week and were fortunate that we could be in such close proximity for a number of reasons, including what happened that night.

I had posted something to Facebook to let people know what happened. I am usually a private person, but I wasn't going to be able to hide this, and I wanted it to come from me rather than secondhand sources. After I posted on Facebook, I did something that was one of the smartest things I did in that darkness: I started to write. I grabbed a legal-size yellow pad and wrote to Denise.

I had so many things I never got to say, and I had always heard how therapeutic writing and journaling during times of grief could be. I never paid attention to it much as it was always so cliché, and frankly when would I have ever been the person to whom this would happen?

I wrote to her and was proud of the words I said to her. I tried to go to sleep, but, as you can imagine, rest was hard to find. I just lay there and, every once in a while, I would check the comments on Facebook and read the love and support people shared. I spent more time on Facebook that night than I probably ever had. Reading all the kind comments filled the endless hours when I needed to stay quiet because we all had a long week ahead of us.

I felt so empty lying there by myself, and I could never fall asleep. It was pretty bad. The few times I managed to nod off were short lived, and I would wake within minutes. I didn't know what to do. About 2:00 a.m. I heard someone get up. I was relieved to find that it was Bill going downstairs because he too couldn't sleep. I went down with him, and we agreed there was no way to sleep with what had happened.

There sitting with Denise's father in the wee hours, I just lost it. I had kept myself together as well as I could around people until then, but I couldn't do it anymore. I cried and wailed and we were all up by this time.

My parents came out of their room. To see me in the state I was in was something that no parent would want. It was what it was, and it was our lives. There was talk about whether or not I needed to get some meds to help me deal with the week ahead. I was adamant that I would not take meds because I didn't want to be cloudy and on drugs when I saw Denise for those last times.

I learned then about the power of crying. After that enormous emotional spell, I felt so exhausted I was able to go upstairs and fall asleep for a bit. We all knew that we wouldn't be able to sleep as much as we needed, and eating was going to be difficult, but we also realized that we had a long week ahead and had to try our best to take care of ourselves. Finally, I was able to get to sleep, ending the worst 24 hours of my life.

As bad as my life was at that moment, it was not going to get better for a long time. I found it impossible to think about how and when things would get better. We were dropped into one of the most unimaginable pains, and there was no end in sight. We were all about to walk a journey that we should have never been on. It was the worst tragedy that we could imagine, and we were going to take that long road together whether we wanted to or not.

Chapter 3

The First Week

The next couple days we all lived through the lowest of lows. We experienced a pain that none of us ever could have imagined. I hated being in the middle but was proud of how well the family came together. It should never take something so horrible to bring us all closer. Sadly, it does. The next morning I couldn't eat but was able to go out for a walk with my dad. After getting back, I attempted to take a shower.

This was my made-for-TV moment. In the shower, I just cried with everything I had and crumpled into the fetal position. As I was lying in an atmosphere of complete sadness, a part of me recognized how cliché this was. I had seen a scene like this a number of times on television and in films but never thought I would live that moment.

I had everything and then it was all gone.

Soon we started getting visitors to the house. One was my good friend Derek. I had known him for a little over ten years. Our paths had crossed on many occasions in a number of different cities.

Derek is a runner and so am I. We both value the ability to get outside, and, as Derek hung around the house a lot that week, there were times when he read the situation as well as anyone could. He was good about speaking up and saying that I needed a walk. I took several walks with Derek that week. None of them were good. I was living the darkest moments of my life and pouring my heart out to Derek about all the emotions that threatened to overwhelm me.

Eventually I noticed that he never cried. I couldn't believe he hadn't broken down with emotion as I shared what I was feeling. I was thankful that he was strong enough to handle the onslaught of emotions I displayed. I truly believe most people wouldn't have been able to listen to some of the things that I said on those walks, but Derek was, and, because of that, I never held back.

As a family, we all had a long week in front of us. We spent the time at Bill and Judy's house. I'm sure it was an inconvenience for them, but I knew they didn't mind about becoming the central location for us to gather. Their little cocker spaniel, Olaf, probably objected though since he spent a large part of that week in the garage.

My parents and I stayed at Bill and Judy's for the week and that became where people came to talk to all of us. Bill, Judy, Dawn, and I created what I called the brain trust. We made many of the important decisions there. We faced a lot of difficult moments, but not everything was bad.

Early on, the investigator dropped by to talk to us. He was the same person who questioned me after Denise's death. He showed professionalism and compassion. The five of us went upstairs and listened to the investigator. He brought us some good news that we all wanted and needed to hear.

He looked at me with kindness as he said, "Based on the information we collected, your wife went quickly and wasn't in pain."

A collective sigh of relief from the group of us followed his words. We all had been afraid she had suffered. I felt terrified that I wouldn't be able to handle if I found out my wife was in pain and I wasn't there for her.

While we were upstairs, we continued to have family and friends arrive to give their condolences. Everyone was caring and respectful. I had a couple friends travel from over an hour away.

Just before they showed up, Dawn and I had been trying to figure out what we would tell people who wanted to give donations. Since Denise didn't really have a disease or an ailment that seemed to be the underlying cause, we didn't have a medical foundation to suggest for donations. We felt it would be in the best interest to look into a 501c3 organization. We really just wanted to designate a nonprofit organization where we could direct people's donations and do some good. We agreed that we could do things that we knew Denise believed in and represented the type of person she was.

My friends from out of town who were there had worked in the banking community. We told them our plan and they hit the phones.

During that period, someone who didn't know better might have thought we were selling drugs. There were various men on cell phones all around the front of the house and cars running down the block. It was a sight to see. It was good to have so many people trying to help. We still didn't know the best way to solve our nonprofit challenge, so Derek, Brian, my father, and I went to our local bank and spoke with them.

The banker with whom we spoke had been good to Denise and me. He had worked with us through setting up our joint checking accounts and all our finances. To hear why we were there was pretty hard for him, I imagine. It all seemed so wrong and the only thing that drove us during that time was to try and find a way to honor Denise.

To make a long story short, a family member established a UCARE page, a friend of Denise's from California worked the phone, and we were able to set up the Denise H. Moore Memorial Fund through the North Carolina Community Foundation. People who wanted to support us now had a way, and we could in turn do something with that money that we felt Denise would have wanted. We were happy about being able to carry on Denise's legacy and thankful to the many people who helped make this happen.

I continued to receive a lot of support from a number of sources including Facebook. Many people whom I hadn't heard from in years reached out. I was still in such shock that I didn't know what to say and wasn't able to respond to most of them. There were really no words. Although I was never particularly good with social media sites, it meant a lot to me that people were reaching out and trying to provide encouragement to all of us in our time of need.

People brought over food and drinks and attempted to support us in any way they could. I couldn't eat anything. I tried to but really couldn't bring myself to put anything in my stomach. Since we were on the go so much that week, I didn't really push myself to eat. I developed stomachaches, but it didn't really match the pain I felt in my heart.

At one point, I did something smart. I needed to put calories in me but didn't want to eat, so I began drinking smoothies and milkshakes to try to keep up my energy level, knowing that I wasn't going to be sitting down and eating many meals. At one point Derek offered to pick up something, and I asked him to just get milkshakes so when I got hungry I would have one. In the way only Derek could, he showed up about a half hour later very excited, saying he had brought us fried chicken and milkshakes. It was a welcomed sight. He was enthusiastic about the chicken, and I had a milkshake and we froze the rest.

One evening while I was out, an unexpected visitor came to Bill and Judy's. The investigator who had been so good to me stopped by with his wife, who had made a turkey tetrazzini dish, and delivered it to the family. I don't know if I ate an actual meal the first three days, but I did eat a fair amount of that. I have no idea why I was able to eat that but I did. All the bagels and breads people were bringing seemed too difficult to swallow. The whole family ate the turkey tetrazzini, and not one of us will forget how good it tasted and how much better we all felt after that meal.

Making arrangements for a funeral is never easy, but our circumstances made it even more difficult. We found a funeral home that was recommended and agreed to use them. We were able to hold the service and the viewing at the church where Bill and Judy attended and Denise and I occasionally visited. We were lucky that the church was so accommodating for us.

As Denise's family and mine sat around a table at the funeral home to talk about the preparations, the situation continued to seem so terribly wrong. Those first couple of days we were constantly in motion, always keeping busy. Sitting around that table was hard. There were going to be some tough decisions, and we all made them as well as we could and together as a family.

We needed to discuss Denise's clothing. One of the most difficult things we had to consider was if there were any clothes she would be able to wear with her being so pregnant. We had to ask the unthinkable question: Were the babies still in Denise or had they been removed? This would determine what she could wear. They told us the babies had been removed, and we agreed to have Denise wear her beautiful dress from the baby shower.

At the end of the meeting we asked if Denise was at the funeral home.

"Yes," the director told us. "If you would like to see her, we have a room you can use."

None of us wanted to see her but we all needed to. I had no idea what I was walking into when I went through those double doors. What I saw was both beautiful and the worst thing I had ever seen in my life. Denise was so lovely. I valued the limited moments I would be able to see her physical body. However, this was not how our lives were supposed to go. Because Denise was so pregnant, they had to tilt her head in a way that caused all her extra skin around her face to fall on her chin.

Denise would have hated the way she looked. She was always self-conscious as we all are. Her extra "pregnant skin" showed because of how she was placed. I loved this woman but looking down on her was so heartbreaking. I could barely stand seeing how she now was.

I could handle being there for only a short time. I was extremely torn during those moments. I knew I wasn't going to be able to see Denise much more before her cremation, but this was not the Denise I knew. It was so difficult for all of us.

I have rarely seen my father sad. And I have never seen him as helpless and pathetic as I did that day. The way he looked at me was heartbreaking. My dad is always so full of life, very much like Denise was. I had never seen him look like that and it was just awful. I felt for him. He was looking at the big picture while, in that moment, I was just feeling Denise's passing.

I love my dad and we have had talks about that moment. It's something that will stick with us for the rest of our lives. I have never seen my dad the way he looked at me that day— such grief and sympathy etched on his features. Seeing Denise like that was a sad reminder for all of us how one minute we had the whole world in front of us and the next it was all gone and destroyed.

Denise was always a warm and loving person, not the cold and distant shell we saw in that room. I will always love her and that moment was no different in that respect. I just wished our ending wouldn't have led us to a funeral home when we should have been in a hospital as proud parents welcoming our babies into the world.

This tragedy touched many lives. Many people with whom Denise and I worked had a hard time with this. I realized I probably should say something to people, but I didn't know how to find the words. I had reached out to Denise's principal as well as my principal to see if they both felt that each school would benefit from me coming in and talking to them. It was such an emotional time for me but also for people who worked with us. Both of our principals knew each other and Denise's principal said that it might be beneficial to come in and talk to Denise's team.

Derek, dad, and I went to the school, and I talked to a couple ladies who were close to Denise. The last time I had seen them was when they came to her baby shower. I talked to them about how I was doing and asked how they were holding up. We spoke for maybe an hour about anything and everything. I didn't feel I handled myself as well as I could have, but I think I was comforting to them. They were having a hard time, and I believe that after I spoke to them they seemed to do a little better. I felt that I might have done a decent job of trying to help them keep their focus on their students while at school. I'm sure it was extremely hard walking past Denise's door every day and trying to stay strong in front of the students.

My principal probably won't admit it, but I believe she was okay with me coming to talk to my school the next day, knowing I didn't buckle in front of Denise's team. If I would have shown up and lost it in front of everyone, I think it easily could have made the situation a lot worse. My dad came with me when I went to my school. My principal had told the staff that I would come in after school if they wanted to stay. Dad and I sat in the principal's office while school let out and then were taken to the library. I had sat in that library more times than I could remember for all our staff meetings, early release meetings, and sadly our school's baby shower. This time

I would be the one talking rather than the one who usually listened.

A large number of teachers and even some of the teacher assistants were there to show their support for me. I walked in and didn't really know what to do or say. I just spoke from my heart. I started off explaining to them that I didn't know what to do or say but that I felt and needed their love and support. I didn't know what the future was going to hold for me. I felt I would try to go back to work, but I had no idea if I was going to be able to.

I was able to stay focused enough to recognize that quite a few people were having a hard time. Tears were being shed and sadness permeated the entire group. I told everyone I would need them now and even more desperately in the future when everyone got back to their lives, and I had to figure out what my life would become without Denise. I finished by telling people that I appreciated them staying and caring for me. I offered them all a hug, and to my surprise everyone stayed and came up to me and gave me a hug.

Being there in front of my peers and talking with them was therapeutic for me. I can't explain it but I felt good about opening up to people. I was in the darkest place of my life, but I knew that people cared enough to let me share my thoughts and feelings, even though my words were clouded in sadness. I appreciated the time they gave me. As all the staff members left and went back to their lives, my father and I headed back to more sadness and our home base for the week.

Earlier in the day, the family and I went to the church to meet with the pastors to talk about the service. We spoke openly about everything. Although Denise and I had attended the church, we didn't really know the pastors. They both wanted

37

to know a little more about us so they could speak about what kind of person Denise was. They seemed professional and personable, and I knew Denise would have liked them.

The next evening was the viewing. It would be the second to last time I would get to see Denise's physical body. In all the chaos of the week, I soon realized that I didn't have any black pants. Denise and I had just recently, within the last three months, moved into our new house. Before the move I threw out my black pants as they were a little short and not worth keeping and packing. Dawn was nice enough to go to Kohl's and get me a couple pairs to wear for the viewing and funeral.

Dawn did a large amount of work that week. We had a lot of discussions about the fund and were together a great deal. We were a really good team. One of Dawn's projects she worked so well on was trying to get a large number of pictures of Denise. She went through a number of phones and computers and got a great deal of Denise though the years. Some pictures were before I came around and many I had never seen before. Once she had them all compiled, she sent them to Brian who had the task of placing them together with music to show as a film during the viewing.

I often went upstairs during those days to find Brian sitting in front of a computer with tears in his eyes, trying to stay focused on his task. The afternoon of the viewing he let me take a look at the film. Both Bill and I sat and watched it. It was beautifully done and lasted about 30 minutes. We both cried a lot. The film, like a lot what happened that week, was both beautiful and heartbreaking. I was so glad I watched it before the viewing because it evoked intense emotions, and I knew I would need to try to keep myself together as best I could for everyone who came through the viewing line. Both Dawn and Brian did an unbelievable job making the film a reality.

The viewing was well organized and put together. We had three tables of items that represented Denise for people to look at. We also had a couple tables of paper and pencils for people to write stories or memories or anything they wanted to share. Denise was extremely crafty, and a couple of her friends did a beautiful job of organizing those tables. Denise would have been proud.

Seeing so many people attend was overwhelming. We were at the church talking to people for about four hours. There was a line out the door and many people waited for multiple hours. A number of people watched the 30-minute film a couple times while they waited. Some visitors weren't even able to see us because the line was so long. There were friends, family, people whom Denise taught, and many of my former students as well. The outpouring of support touched us deeply, and it felt so good to know that people cared, that this affected their lives. Some traveled from out of state because they wanted to be there. The captain of the local police department was there along with people who used to work with Denise whom I had never met. The large attendance was a testament to how wonderful Denise was. It was a long night and by the time it all ended, my back was really sore from bending over so many times. But it was a good pain because I knew that people cared and that Denise was well loved. That night I was exhausted and slept okay with some help from medication, but I knew that the next day was going to be the most difficult.

We held the funeral at the same church the next afternoon. They let us see Denise one more time before they closed the casket.

I would never see the love of my life again.

I managed to walk less than halfway down the aisle before my emotions got the best of me. It was so hard and horrible. I just wanted us to have the life we should have had. This was one of the most depressing and emotional times of the week.

There had been a lot of talk about who would speak at the funeral. We got a couple of Denise's closest friends, and her principal agreed to say something. As they were giving their speeches, I realized they were much better writers than I was and that my letter was far shorter than theirs.

We had a number of conversations that week about whether I should get up and talk. I hadn't been involved in too many funerals, so I didn't really know the custom of whether someone so close to the loved one should say something. I was pretty adamant that I would say something.

For the last couple of evenings, I worked on my letter to Denise, and, while we were waiting for the funeral to start, I sat outside and read over my writing as much as I could. I wasn't sure how I would handle reading in front of everyone but felt I needed to know what I'd written as best I could.

As I sat there in front of the casket, I watched the pallbearers. I watched as my friend Derek, who had been there for me that week through my deep sadness and had managed to stay strong for me, finally get tears in his eyes. I was amazed but not surprised. This kind of sadness is not something we are built for. When it was my turn to speak, I walked up and looked out at the audience.

The school district made an amazing gesture. As the funeral was held during school hours, all the neighboring schools pulled together and tried to get coverage for anyone that wanted to come and show their support. I heard stories from people who didn't even know us, who traveled to either Denise or my school, just to cover the class for someone that wanted to be there. We reserved a whole side of the sanctuary for teachers and school personnel as we knew they might get in a little late because they were traveling from work. Their entire section was filled by the start of the funeral. I saw a number of people whom Denise and I knew, and I felt honored that I worked in a county that would make the effort to do something for us in our most desperate time of need.

I spoke from my heart and read from my paper. I wanted to look up and show people my face. It was really hard and I focused on making it the way it should be. There was one point when I was on the verge of breaking down, and I felt the pastor put his hand on my back, and I was able to keep it together. I don't know if I will ever speak more impactfully than I did that day. I was so glad my letter was short because I was able to make it through. I focused so intently that as I walked off the stage I almost missed the first step. If I would have tumbled down the stairs, I would have ended up in the fetal position, crying right there in front of everyone. Luckily I caught myself and was able to avoid a scene.

The service was as good as it could be. The pastor told a story about Denise and me on our first date. We had been waiting before a movie and were sitting on a bench watching all these unsupervised kids running around on this patch of grass. I turned to her and jokingly said, "You know we could take one of them and no one would know."

It was a funny little anecdote that made people smile a bit. This wasn't the ideal closing for the service, but under the circumstances it was the fitting ending.

As we walked Denise's coffin out and loaded her into the hearse, we could feel the warmth from the sunlight on our faces, which made it so much more real. I stood by myself as the vehicle drove away.

That day was the last time I was ever able to see Denise, and it seemed that this world would forever be much darker. As the hearse traveled away to the point I could no longer see it, I knew that I would never be the same. As the vehicle drove away, so did the life Denise and I built. She took a large part of my heart with her. The life we worked so hard for had departed.

She was so beautiful. She always treated this world better than it treated her. She deserved so much more, and her life was cut far too short.

Being a mother was all she ever wanted. Yes, we can say that she is one in Heaven with our twins, but the sad reality of it was that she would have been an amazing mother to those beautiful children here on Earth, and she never got the chance. Sadly, the world and I would never get to see the joy those children would have brought to her.

Chapter 4

Returning to Work

With all the family and friends in town and the funeral just over, we all gathered outside the new home I had shared with Denise. Most of those present hadn't been to the new house before Denise's passing, so it was good they came over and got to see the outside of it.

My parents bought some light blue, pink, and white balloons to represent Denise and the two babies. We passed out a balloon to everyone as we assembled in front of the house. Having them there with me touched my heart. I said a couple words and we let the balloons go. Not all of them went up in the air but most did. It was a sweet and difficult moment. As surely the air currents carried away those balloons, the lives of my loving wife and unborn babies left us.

The kids who were there chased after some of the balloons that didn't fly, which lightened the mood. The family thought releasing the balloons would be a helpful symbolic gesture, and we all agreed it went well even if a few of the balloons failed to rise to the sky.

After the ceremony, everyone headed to lunch at Bill and Judy's house. Being together was meaningful even though none of us wanted to be there. It's sad that often times it takes something like this to get everyone together. Given the tragic circumstances, I believe we needed to be together to heal. I met some of Denise's family whom I had never seen and others to whom I was introduced at our wedding. It went as well as it could have. Our principals came over to the house as well, which was kind of them.

There were people who I hadn't seen on my side of the family who I hadn't been able to talk to in person since the wedding. It was nice to talk to them but somehow much of our conversation geared toward the on-slot of sadness that this week was and what I would be up against going forward.

While talking to people, I managed to speak rationally and was proud of how well I handled everything. Bill and Judy understandably continued to struggle, but they opened their house to the large group and acted as loving hosts. As people began to leave, we tried to clean up as best we could. A couple family members were going to stay for another day or two, but the reason they came into town was behind us.

Many of us were filled with such love and support that at the time we felt we were doing okay. However, as people systematically left, we all knew the outpouring of love would soon end. We were grateful that so many people had taken time out of their lives to be a part of ours when we needed them the most. But this loss was going to be forever with us.

The sad truth was that the buildup to the funeral had taken some of our focus, and now we had to face the sadness. With the funeral behind us, family and friends had to return to their own lives, and there were no more distractions from the ever-present grief.

I stayed at Bill and Judy's for a few more days as my parents transitioned back into the house Denise and I built for our future. My parents had the painful job of taking all the baby things that were spread all over the house and putting them into the nursery. I knew that would be extremely difficult, but, as my parents pointed out, it was only one small piece of what we would have to deal with in the coming weeks and months.

Within a few days, I went back into the house. By then, Mom had headed back to Tennessee, and Dad was going to stay with me for much longer as we navigated through the uncharted challenges of this heavy loss.

I couldn't bring myself to sleep in our bed, so Dad was nice enough to let me take the guest bedroom while he slept on the couch. I felt bad putting him on the sofa, but there weren't many other options in the house, and I knew that Dad didn't mind.

We spent some time walking during the days and trying to figure out all the things that we were going to need to do. It was going to be difficult, and I had to keep active and moving to avoid being overwhelmed by my sadness. Luckily a lot of people seemed to empathize with what I was going through and sent cards and support. I heard from many friends and had a bunch of thank-you cards to write. I took great care to thank the many who had sent money, which I collected and put toward the fund we had set up in Denise's memory. That seemed to be the best use of the money.

I was fortunate that my family covered the cost of the funeral. Not everyone has that kind of assistance. A lot of people have to rely heavily on donations to try to cover the overwhelming financial cost of a funeral. Since I didn't have to worry about that, I was able to deposit a good amount of money into the fund and write thank-you cards for all the people who showed their support.

Writing those notes gave me a sense of purpose for a while. It also showed me how many people's lives had been touched, and it was nice to know that people cared. Writing the cards was a good way for me to clean up a small part of the house and also serve as a small bit of therapy in the words that I wrote.

I began making phone calls to places I knew would need to know about Denise's passing. Over the last couple of months, Denise and I had consolidated our money into one bank account so we could work on our budget and save enough to pay Bill and Judy for watching our twins. As a result, I knew the money that was going out and was able to reach out to places like the companies that held Denise's school loans and talk to them about the situation.

Having Dad there helped since a lot of the things I was having to do were far beyond my ability level. Just understanding everything was pretty challenging. We were given the name of an estate lawyer and met with her, which seemed to be the best way to handle a lot of the issues that arose. We also stopped by banks, did some online research, and followed up on the fallout from Denise's passing.

I hated everything we were having to do, but the more active I was, the less I thought about my sadness. If I sat still for too long, the grief that lay just beneath the surface would rise and overwhelm me. I let go and cried each day in the shower. Dad soon learned that there were always going to be times when I would get emotional, but, with so much to do, we tried to keep ourselves as busy as we could. I attempted to go to the gym to get back into some kind of routine, hoping that would ease my emotional state.

"Mom and I think it would be good for you to try to go back to work," Dad said one day.

I felt like I didn't have anything else to do during the day but didn't know if it would be healthy to go in and had no idea how to act. I also feared that I wouldn't be able to keep myself together to help the kids I worked with daily.

My mom remained hopeful that I could go back to work. She understood that I needed structure and also the distraction from what my life had become. I wasn't ready to return to teaching yet. Dad and I stayed busy that week after the funeral. Many tasks still loomed over me. However, the seed had been planted. Returning to school would become one of my first main hurdles.

Dad and I took the two weeks following the funeral to get as much done as we could. After we took care of the largest issues, most of what remained would be handled through the estate lawyers, and that required little from me.

Because I wasn't going to work for a while, I stayed up late and watched TV. Although neither my father nor I are night owls, we wanted to watch Denise's favorite team, the Chicago Cubs, in the World Series. We saw the Cubs win the World Series. It was a touching moment. I couldn't tell you the last time Dad and I watched a baseball game together before that. We were both happy for the Cubs and glad to know that Denise would have been really pleased.

As busy as I kept myself, there were still things I needed to deal with. The twins were supposed to be born on October 31, and I wanted to honor them somehow on that day. I hoped to do something that I could repeat every year to always remind me of those kids I never got to meet. Their due date being on Halloween was a really hard pill to swallow. As Dad and I walked around the neighborhood and saw all the Halloween decorations, we felt uneasy. It felt odd and uncomfortable seeing all those fake tombstones when Denise and the twins had just passed.

On October 31, Bill, Judy, my Dad, and I, went to a park and walked around a lake. I felt this was something Denise and I would have enjoyed doing with the children. Afterward, we went to get ice cream, which was another thing Denise and I would have done with the kids. I ordered my sherbet and I got Denise her sweet and salty flavored ice cream. Her ice cream sadly went uneaten.

It was probably the best way to start a tradition that I hoped to carry on in some form or another for the rest of my life to always remember the lives and future that we all lost.

I wasn't sure about passing out candy on Halloween. It was another tough decision I had to make. I knew Denise would want me to give candy to the kids. Both of us always enjoyed sitting on the front porch, handing out treats and seeing all of the costumes.

In times like these, you see the best in people. I witnessed this myself. The investigator whose job it was to make sure I didn't have anything to do with Denise's passing had asked if he could come over and sit with me and pass out candy. It was an amazing gesture and, sure enough, the two of us and my dad sat out on my front porch and handed out treats.

It made me feel good that someone whom I had met in the worst moment of my life identified the struggle I was facing and agreed to come and give his time to be with me. I have always felt there should be more stories of people offering such kindnesses.

With October behind me, it was time to start thinking about how I could transition back into the real world. I really didn't want to start but realized it was a step in the right direction. I had spent a good amount of time at my principal's house, which was only a couple blocks away. We had talked about my students and which ones needed to know about the passing of Denise and the twins.

Many of my students were aware of Denise's pregnancy, and, because we were so close to her delivery date, the assumption would have been that I hadn't started back to school because Denise had the babies and all was right with the world. The school took the names of the families to whom I was closest and contacted them to let them know the sad news. I wasn't privy to how those conversations went, but I imagine those parents with whom I had been close for years probably had a difficult time hearing about what happened.

My students were one of the few bright spots in my life after Denise died. As a special education teacher, I get to work with kids for multiple years, and often I develop close relationships with them and their families. The students I served that year had been in my class for a couple years.

When I first came to the school, I taught mainly first and fifth graders. That year my fifth graders included my amazing student Davis, whom I will always feel I was meant to teach. When Davis' group left, I kept the first graders and followed them all the way through their fifth grade.

While I was unsure about being ready to go back to work, I knew without a doubt that I was ready to be with my kids. After the talks with my wonderful principal, I recognized that my biggest issue was not going to be the returning to teaching but keeping up with all the paperwork. Teaching special education is a blessing and a curse. The blessing is you have a great set of students, but the downside is the amount of paperwork required in the limited amount of time that you aren't teaching.

With my ever-changing view of the world, I could only see the big picture. Being a teacher is first and foremost about the students and the interactions with the kids. Sitting at the computer and filling out a bunch of forms on students that you may or may not teach definitely is a less important aspect of the job. Even when Denise was living, the amount of paperwork I had was overwhelming and often produced a great deal of frustration when I felt the amount of paperwork diminished my time for instruction and pulled my focus away from giving the kids the very best I could. They usually gave me their very best and they deserved at least that much from me.

As I expressed my concerns to my principal, she was considerate and understanding. She knew my passion for my kids. Also, I think she recognized that returning to teaching was a stepping stone in my life. She did a great job of taking her principal hat off and putting her compassion hat on. The other two special education teachers with whom I worked agreed to hold my meetings for me, which was an amazing gesture. With so much negativity in my life, knowing that I could go to school and just teach gave me such a sense of relief. It was probably the best way to handle this unique transition.

I asked my principal to let the other teachers know I was unlikely to feel up to chatting after my return and would need to keep to myself. I believe my principal and the whole staff were ready for me to attempt to come back to school. We understood that I might not be able to cope, and, if I needed to take a leave of absence, that was always an option. However, I knew it was something I had to at least try. So three weeks after my whole world came crashing down, I attempted to resume my professional career and rejoin the work force.

The first morning was tough. I had been used to staying in bed as long as I could because sleep was still scarce for me even with my medication. Waking up early that first day proved difficult. I didn't have as much time to cry in the shower as I usually had. However, I was excited to see my students, but nervous about how people would treat me. I worried that I would not handle things as well as I had previously.

I always prided myself on my way with students. However, working with them was easier done when I was happy. Now I was navigating intense emotions and wasn't sure how patiently I could handle all aspects of teaching.

When I arrived at work, I used a side entrance and tried to keep my head low. I saw a couple people, but I had no idea what to say to anyone, so I just tried to get into the classroom and get my mind right for my kids. Upon entering, I discovered that a couple of thoughtful staff members had left me some Diet Mountain Dew and an eight-pack of my favorite G2 flavor, raspberry lemonade. It was a kind gesture that almost made me smile.

As the students arrived, I fell into my teaching routine and many of the kids did a really good job of just doing what I have always asked of them in my class. I had a number of students come up and give me a hug and one of my newer ones gave me a teddy bear, which was an incredibly sweet gesture. As the day progressed, I was pleased with how I handled myself and how everyone at school, staff members and students, treated me. Driving home I felt exhausted but was proud that I made it through the first day.

The following day was not as successful. I soon realized that I built up the first day so much in my head that I totally forgot that it was the beginning of a string of days that would continue throughout the school year. That second day I felt completely empty and didn't seem to be able to get my head back into teaching. I was going through the motions, but I didn't have the heart for it. It was odd and sad. I felt disappointed in myself because I have always believed I should work for my kids as hard as they work for me. That day I wasn't able to live up to that standard, but I also understood that every day was going to be a strange rollercoaster of emotions.

Having a bad second day was tough, but I learned that not every day would be decent. I realized I simply had to face what every day would bring. Day three went better and soon I was able to keep myself together fairly well. I learned quickly that I didn't need to talk to staff in the hallway before school, but the more I interacted with my students, the more I got caught up in my professional life and almost forgot about my personal tragedy. The students were good for me, and, although everything wasn't perfect at school, work brought something positive into my life, which I badly needed.

It was also helpful that I was still able to come home to someone at the house. Dad was still staying with me, and, as the year went on, both my parents did a good job of visiting me and helping me with the emptiness and loneliness I was feeling. Those first few days at school were wearing, but being able to come home and walk and talk with my dad eased my tensions and helped me release of a lot of emotions.

I fell into a groove of trying not to look at people before school and getting to my classroom as quickly as I could. The more I interacted with other staff members, the worse I felt. I can't explain it, but many of the adults soon realized that I wasn't good at the beginning of school, but, as the day progressed, I slowly returned to the person I used to be at work. The students often brought the best out of me. With what I was going through, they were the best things I had in my life.

As I continued with work, I still felt miserable when I was in the room by myself. I had all these emotions and questions in my head that often made teaching hard. I ended up finding a couple staff members who didn't have morning duties and just essentially dumped my sadness on them. I felt bad about doing it, but we all understood that the more I talked, the less pent-up emotion I had to hold and the more I mentally was able to get ready for the daily instruction. I referred to it as "drying up the well." I tried hard to clean the tears out of my eyes by the time the students showed up in class, but I wasn't always successful. With their support, I was able to find a better balance of my emotional state so I could give those students my best.

The paperwork aspect of my job is extremely demanding. I felt sorry that the other two special education teachers, who already had a heavy load of paperwork, had to handle even more. Most situations where work and this kind of tragedy intersect aren't handled as well as this. While my students helped to draw my focus out of the pain I felt, I would be remiss if I didn't express how much I appreciated what the other special education teachers did for my mental state. In taking over my administrative responsibilities, I could do the job of simply being a special education teacher to the best of my abilities.

I still had an incredibly long journey ahead of me. Facing challenges is often referred to as an uphill climb. I quickly realized for me this was more like a mountain range than a hill. Going back to work was the first small mountain I had to scale. The journey forward was going to take a great deal of time and countless tears. But the outlet of teaching helped me reintegrate into a world that didn't make any sense to me.

Chapter 5

Restless

My parents traded off with each other in order to spend time with me. During those few weeks of going back to work, I felt grateful to come home to someone. I spent only a few days, perhaps about a week, by myself. I had taken for granted the joy I'd experienced coming home to be with Denise each day. Without her, loneliness and sorrow were my only companions on the drive home. My parents' presence at the house during that difficult time made the transition from my professional life to my personal life a little easier.

I was able to go to the gym in the mornings and come directly home after school most days, which made it much easier to stay focused on my students. I was thankful to have an eight-hour distraction from whatever my life had become.

Early in the period after my return to work, I began to realize a few things. The first was something with which I always struggled but now was worse than ever. I have Attention Deficit Hyperactivity Disorder (ADHD), so I am usually busy. As an adult having ADHD is actually a blessing in some ways. I have a lot of energy but need to find outlets to direct it. Denise and I were a well-suited team; she cooked the dinners and I cleaned afterward. Between work and the limited housework I did in the evenings, I released a fair amount of my energy. After I cleaned up, we often just hung out on the couch and watched a movie or TV show.

After her death I wasn't able to relax as I had with Denise. I walked with my parents, but, even after returning and eating dinner, I just couldn't manage to sit in front of the television.

My head was constantly running and many of the emotions and thoughts flowing through my head weren't positive ones. I was lucky enough to find an outlet that not only helped me through those evenings but also became a form of therapy for me.

While Denise was alive, I found myself occasionally playing with Legos. I had got a Lego architecture set somewhere and enjoyed putting it together. For those who are unaware, these sets are essentially Legos for fully functioning adults. The Lego Company created sets based on famous structures or houses with the correct pieces that people like me could construct. I had done about three of these while Denise and I watched football before her passing, and I enjoyed building them. After Denise's passing, I bought one just to give me something to do and to keep me engaged. I soon found that all I wanted to do in the evenings was to come home and work on Legos.

I always heard that during times of stress people often resort to things they liked as a child, and, as I moved through this sadness, I guess I did the same thing.

I discerned that I needed to rest my body after work since keeping myself together continued to be a full-time job. However, I couldn't bring myself to sit still for longer than 15 minutes.

Legos became my therapy. I bought a couple of sets when I went into Raleigh. One of my purchases happened when my father and I went to where Denise and I had bought our rings. I wanted to make Denise's wedding ring into a necklace. Upon arriving an employee came to talk to me. She looked at my face and saw that I was an emotional wreck and was nice enough to help me put the wedding ring on the necklace. The company did it for free, which says a lot about this company because I would have paid a good chunk of money for what it meant to me.

While my dad and I got that done, I bought a Lego set and once I got home there wasn't much else I wanted to do. I just started building.

I quickly found myself constructing with Legos most weekends and building after I got home from work and whenever else I could. I literally felt compelled to be active, and this became a way for me to waste away the evenings and escape the emptiness. My parents made dinner and then let me go straight to the Legos while they cleaned up. Legos provided a process to work through from beginning, to middle, to the final finished product.

The greater meaning behind this activity still escapes me, but I do know that it gave me something to look forward to while I drove home from work to my sad life. Many days and evenings I sat in the dining room and worked on Legos. I got to the point where I could put together sets pretty quickly, and I needed to have enough of them to keep me busy and my mind occupied. I bought a number of sets on Amazon. There were a couple days when I didn't have any, and I had no idea what to do with myself. Luckily those days were few and far between as the next day a set or two would show up. I enjoyed the bigger projects that took multiple days; I really took pride in them. It was a childish toy that I used to help me get through a horrendous time.

When I first started putting together Legos, I listened to music while I worked on each set. All the melody-filled songs I played seemed mournful and were anything but upbeat. I made a playlist of about eight songs and listened to them over and over.

It took a couple months to get to the point where I could listen to more upbeat music to keep my brain active. It was a unique time. I was fortunate the money I used on getting over Denise's passing was spent of Legos rather than drugs or alcohol.

I continued to have a hard time looking at people before school, but as the day progressed I became more social. In the weeks after all Denise died, it took a good while for me to respond to anyone whether through text message or voicemails. I had no idea what to say to people.

There was one teacher from work, Ms. Davenport, who did this really great thing a couple weeks after Denise's passing. She sent me jokes. I didn't respond to them, but it was something

Dad and I would talk about. At one point she sent me a joke, and I actually replied that I thought the joke was funny.

This was probably the first text message or call I made to anyone outside the family. This gave her an opening to ask how I was doing, and I said I was surviving and that Dad was helping me through it. She asked if she and another of the teachers at school could bring over dinner some night. I didn't know how to answer as I was still closed with a lot of people. I didn't have anything to say to anybody and I liked it that way. However, Ms. Davenport had been working so hard in trying to keep me upbeat. I knew I needed to start to let people in, and she would be the type of person around whom I could feel comfortable.

Very soon after I agreed, Ms. Davenport and another teacher, Ms. Gillespie, came over and had dinner with Dad and me. They were reserved when they walked in as I expected them to be. Up until this point, not too many people had seen me apart from talking to the staff a couple days after the passing. We talked about school and how I was doing and it felt good to be social again. My dad is a talker and in those moments when I didn't have anything to say, he did a good job of keeping the conversation going. The dinner was delicious, the company was good, and the evening was beneficial for a couple other reasons.

First, Ms. Davenport said that others at school wanted to help out and that she wanted to know if they could start a dinner list. She asked if people could sign up to bring food over once or twice a week. At the time I still found being around people difficult, but Dad was there and I knew he would help make things easier. If I was having a bad night, I could just accept their food and not talk. I agreed to the idea of the dinner list a couple days a week. Dad and I felt it would be a step in the right direction, and not having to think about dinners would be valuable.

The most important benefit was having people in the house. The house is beautiful and it was Denise's home. I really wanted to share it with people, and luckily Ms. Davenport and Ms. Gillespie were nice enough to let me give them a tour of our palace. As you would expect, going into the nursery was incredibly difficult, but having people to show the house to forced me to walk into that room.

After I agreed to be given dinner assistance, Dad and I were thankful to have food coming a couple times a week. Occasionally we even found ourselves making jokes about how uncomfortable we could make it for the people coming over. These were stupid jests but, seeing as how there wasn't much to laugh about, it was at least something that brought a smile. Dad enjoyed the meals and the dinners turned out to be helpful for both of us.

Between my Legos and the dinners, I soon fell into a routine. I would work and then come home and clean up a little bit before sitting at the dining room table and doing Legos before the dinner arrived or until either Mom or Dad prepared the evening meal. There were a couple times when I invited the people who signed up for that evening's dinner to eat with us. On other occasions, I simply received the food and cooking instructions and said, "Thank you." My emotions were still all over the place, but it was a kind gesture that the school did for me and a step forward in my healing.

By doing the Lego projects so often, I was running out of sets to complete. I had to start buying sets that were rather pricey and discontinued. I didn't mind spending the money because I figured that most people in my situation would spend their money on drugs and alcohol, and I just spent mine on childhood puzzles.

About this time, my wonderful neighbor stopped by to see how I was doing and to talk to me. His name is Adam and he is a kind, genuine guy. He took an interest in all my completed Lego sets. He was probably one of the few people that December who discerned how deeply depressed I was. My parents had gone back to Tennessee and I was all alone. Adam understood when I told him that I wasn't worried about how bad the holidays would be; I was more concerned about just making it to Christmas.

I managed to get through Thanksgiving with Denise's family, and, apart from Bill getting sick and not being able to be with the family, we all did well. It was the first real family holiday without Denise. We made it through together. It was really odd. The empty seat where Denise should have been went unmentioned. We were determined to support each other during this really tough time. We all handled Thanksgiving as well as we could have under the circumstances, but the struggle that Christmas would bring loomed over of us.

Denise's family and I agreed the best way to handle Christmas was to go somewhere. After a lot of discussion, we decided a cruise to some place warm seemed like the best way to handle the catastrophe that Christmas was going to bring this year. We originally planned to leave a couple of days before Christmas, but then we made the smart decision to leave a day after the holiday. The benefit of waiting was that Sara could open her presents at Dawn and Brian's house on Christmas morning. Denise would have wanted it that way.

Even with plans in place, I still struggled with the build-up to Christmas. My anxiety remained high and I was running low on Lego sets to keep me occupied. I just tried to hold on. One afternoon a couple weeks before Christmas, Adam asked me to come to his house. Again, anyone who meets him knows that his true character is that of a great, genuine person. He had done a good job of checking on me, so whatever he needed I would be more than happy to oblige.

Adam and his wife Tricia had gotten six presents for me. I told him he didn't need to do that. Adam, of course, implied that he knew but wanted to get them anyway. He had bought me five different Lego sets. But because I had been completing so many, I already had about half of them.

It touched me that someone went so far out of his way to help me get through the horrible holiday season. When he asked if I had any of those Lego sets, I told him which ones I had and emphasized how excited I was about building the new ones. He went so far as to get find out which ones Bill and Judy planned to give me as Christmas presents so he didn't duplicate their presents. It was an unbelievable gesture. I felt so cared for and deeply appreciative.

Adam said he was going to try to sell the ones I already had, and I felt bad that he went through all that trouble. However, Adam seemed to not really care and just wanted to do something nice for me.

I had totally forgotten that I had mentioned to him that I would have to buy my own presents that year. We planned our normal Christmas tradition with Denise's family, but I would miss having presents at the house. Adam understood this and decided to include me in their holiday. In addition to the Lego sets, he gave me the first nine seasons of his favorite show,

The Big Bang Theory, on DVD. He was aware that I had never seen the show and asked me to give it a shot. I told him I would.

I left his house feeling grateful that someone who cared about me lived so close. Adam understood the daily struggle I was experiencing. I was fortunate to have a neighbor who was thoughtful and concerned with my wellbeing.

I was excited about doing the new Lego sets but wasn't sure I could manage to sit in front of the TV to watch the DVDs. My parents continued to take turns visiting, and my mom was staying with me at this point. She had mentioned that she enjoyed *The Big Bang Theory*, so, although I have never been too excited about network television programming and often found the jokes predictable and plots unengaging, I was willing to watch at least one show with her.

I was pretty skeptical as I've been burned by network television so often, but this show was different, and I can actually say I enjoyed it. I was glad of that for a number of reasons. The main one was that for the first time I had a reason to sit in front of the TV and watch something.

It doesn't seem like that should be that big of a deal, but for me it was. I did some type of exercise every morning, taught, and then came home and did Legos day after day after day. I just kept wearing my body down, and I hardly ever had my anxiety under control enough to relax. Because I couldn't stay still, I kept feeling less than 100% healthy. I never got totally sick, but I spent a fair amount of time during those couple of months feeling unwell because I was failing to rest my body.

I've always felt uncomfortable when I wasn't able to give my students the best I could. Denise understood this, and now because I couldn't sit still I had a tough time trying to be at my best for those students. Finding enjoyment in a TV show allowed me to let go and gave my body and mind a chance for peace. I looked forward to watching nine seasons of the program. I did a much better job of letting my body calm down enough in the evening, which meant I would be less tired for my students the next day.

I was still taking sleep meds every night. They knocked me out when I was ready for bed. I didn't really like having to take the medication, but I already had enough on my plate to worry about before I considered reducing the sleep aid.

At the holiday break from school, I realized I would have a hard time without the structure of the classroom and the gift of my students. On the last day with my kids as I was leaving work, I barely made it to my car before I started breaking down. I fumbled with the keys, trying to see through the tears welling in my eyes. I finally managed to get in the car and just sat there crying.

The kids and the work atmosphere were so good for me, and the structure of the job allowed me to focus and stay centered. I knew the thin veneer of composure would come apart after work. I finally got myself together and headed home.

The next day was a teacher workday, and Mom was able to come to school with me. Again I started crying walking back out to the car because I was losing my daily structure and routine. I wished I could skip Christmas that year, but sadly I couldn't make that happen. My fellow teachers would go to be with their families, but the family Denise and I had planned to build was gone forever.

I was grateful to have Mom with me for a few more days. Her presence couldn't fill the emptiness or make the sadness go away, but her being there made my life less lonely and gave me some solace.

Before Christmas arrived I got a knock on the door. My friendly neighbor Adam, grinning widely, stood there holding a big wrapped package. After I invited him in, he said he had one last thing for me. I was pretty sure I knew what it was. Adam often asked me about the Lego sets that I didn't have, and I showed him the most expensive one that I planned to buy at some point.

By the size of the package, I had a feeling the gift was going to be the Robie House, a Frank Lloyd Wright design. Sure enough I was correct. I told Adam that I couldn't accept it. I knew how much money that set cost. He assured me that it wasn't as expensive as I had seen it go for and that he had actually made a little money when he sold back the Lego sets that I already owned.

"This means so much to me," I said. I didn't have words to express how much his kindness touched me.

"Tricia and I just wanted to do something nice for you," he said. "This one should keep you busy for quite a while."

That was what made this gift so meaningful. Adam recognized my need to stay busy, to focus on something beyond my grief. His actions and many kindnesses reminded me that there are really good people in the world. I needed to think of people like Adam and Tricia in the midst of my current life situation. Their thoughtfulness kept me moving forward, which is something I will never forget.

My mom left with three more days until Christmas. After losing my wife and two babies, I would have preferred to ignore this season focused on family. I wanted to avoid those holiday television commercials that featured happy families. The time away from my kids at school left me feeling at loose ends. I ached for things to go back to normal. But they never would.

I had to keep busy to relieve the endless stream of sorrow. So instead of the joy of our babies' first Christmas, I would concentrate on the massive Lego project until Denise's family and I went on the cruise.

Everyone around me was occupied with their own lives while I tried to figure out how to do deal with the emptiness in the worst time of my life. I was lucky to have made it this far.

Denise's family and I kept to the holiday traditions and had as nice of a time as we could at our yearly Christmas Eve get-together. We gathered at Bill and Judy's house, ate dinner, opened presents and tried to keep ourselves from falling apart. We did well while we were together. However, this year when it was all over, I went home to an empty house, one that was meant for joy and was turning into a place of hopelessness.

Chapter 6

Christmas

Coming home Christmas Eve was really tough. They say that every day things get a little easier. I was on the verge of discovering that statements like that are inaccurate and inappropriate.

I put some of my Christmas Eve presents away and got ready for bed. After I took my sleeping pill, I read whatever grief book I had and fell asleep. I woke up the next morning and got ready to head over to see Sara open her presents. I had decided not to ride with Bill and Judy because I had a sad stop to make first.

Walking up to the church on Christmas morning, I must have looked like a shell of a man. This place that is usually reserved for uplifting people and giving praise to God that morning had a very different feel.

When Denise passed away, I was so heartbroken but knew I had to carry out her wishes. I told the family how Denise and I had discussed that we both wanted to be cremated someday. We spoke only once about this. We were too young to have that kind of conversation and believed we wouldn't have to deal with this topic until well after our children went to college and we had lived a long, full life. But I was thankful the discussion came up that one time.

The family and I decided to have Denise cremated and to place her urn at the church where Bill, Judy, and I attended regularly on Sunday mornings. They had treated us so well. It was painful plodding up that walkway to see Denise that day. Her urn was located in a columbarium, which is a lovely term for an urn locker. This resting place offered a beautiful setting for whatever it's worth.

As I did every Sunday, I sat there and cried that Christmas morning. I read their names, Denise, Addison, and Lucas, my family who died. Everywhere else people were with their loved ones in a much different setting. I usually wept when I went to visit her urn, but this time I felt so much emptier than I could have imagined. Sadness is a paltry word to describe my feelings as I sat there that morning. I spoke to Denise and poured my heart out to her. I told her that we had a good time as a family the night before. I felt she would be proud to know that we continued the family tradition. I held onto that thought.

Denise was a beautiful person inside and outside. Her amazing smile always melted my heart. Come Thanksgiving when Denise was alive, her smile became even brighter. She loved Christmas and both getting and giving presents. She delighted in the atmosphere of the holiday season, and, because she was such a giving person, she always went way above and beyond what many people do. She treasured those details and that made Christmas with her special. Putting up the Christmas tree brought joy to her heart. I loved to watch her carefully placing all of her ornaments on our tree. I learned early on that my place was on the couch when it came time to decorate the tree.

Sitting there in front of her resting place on what was her favorite day of the year seemed so wrong. I was getting used to feeling the anguish, but today it threatened to swallow any hint of joy. The holiday season is a terrible time for those grieving. As I sat there in front of her niche (columbarium plot), I knew I had to pull myself together. I told her and the kids I loved them then headed over to see Sara.

Upon arriving at their house, I felt the intense sadness start to overwhelm me again. I didn't want to cry in front of Sara, and I needed to do my part in getting through today as best as we all could. Sara is a warm, sweet kid, and I wanted her to enjoy the day.

Being an only child with two sets of grandparents, Sara often got spoiled at Christmas. This year was no exception. I watched Sara open her presents, and, after my crying spell in the car before entering, I kept my composure for the most part. I was proud of myself and of the family for giving Sara the best Christmas possible under the circumstances.

After Sara had opened her gifts, I hugged everyone and headed home. I saw few cars on the road and surmised that most people were with their families. I took no comfort in the thought. When I arrived home, I looked at the few unwrapped presents I had bought for Denise including a Chicago Cubs World Series T-shirt and a DVD of the movie *Me Before You*, which she and I had watched about a month before her passing. Denise had read the book and liked the author. I also had gotten her the movie *Pitch Perfect*, a movie we always had fun watching together. This was the third copy of the movie I had purchased for her as the other two had been lent out to others who never returned it, so that was a running joke between us. The presents in the living room chair were reminders of the fact that I would never see Denise open presents again and there would never be more presents under our tree.

A small stuffed bear that a student had given me on the first day of school after the tragedy joined the presents. These items served as a sad reminder of everything that had been lost when Denise died. We had been so happy, we had everything we hoped for, and it was all taken from us at the prime of our lives.

I finally went upstairs. The shower has been a really hard place for me since Denise's passing. When I was at the house, I seemed to be constantly doing something. I always tried to watch movies, read books, or listen to music or podcasts to keep my brain engaged. The more fully occupied my brain was the less time I had to think about the things that made me sad. However, in the shower I was stripped, literally and metaphorically, of all of those distractions. I stood there alone with my thoughts. It was the one place where the reality of the situation caught up to me, reminding me of the sadness that consumed me.

With the water pouring over me that Christmas day, I felt the worst I had since the funeral. I instantly remembered that suicide rates go up around the holidays and I realized why. It was so God awful. I couldn't believe that desolation, that I didn't even see the emptiness coming.

If there was a day I could have ended my life and been reunited with Denise, Addison, and Lucas, it was that day. The raw emotions were uncontrollable. I felt deep empathy for anyone who lost a loved one and understood how painful the holidays are for those people. Trying to put into words the amount of sorrow that I felt that day as the water hit my body, I can say only that it was almost too much to bear.

I figured the holiday season would crush me, but I was blindsided by the intensity of my feelings. I just hung my head and cried. I finally grasped that I just needed to get out as soon as I could and find some way to draw my attention away from the pain, so I washed up as best as I could and got out, immediately putting on my earbuds. I knew I had been through the worst of the day. I just had to make it a few more hours until the family and I headed out of town.

I put my clothes on, grabbed my packed bags, brought them downstairs, and continued working on the Lego set that Adam had given me. I sat there listening to music, trying to pretend that this wasn't Christmas and that everything would be all right. After a while, I got a call from a friend of mine who talked to me about the next big project that I would tackle after the holidays. We discussed the possibility of him helping me set up a 5K race with proceeds going to the memorial fund. He gave me some ideas to consider and said he would help in any way he could. I thanked him for his time.

He couldn't have known what his call meant to me on the hardest holiday I will ever have. He was a good friend, something I desperately needed with the level of sadness I held inside me then.

When Bill and Judy came to pick me up, I put my bags in the car and we traveled to Florida. It felt good to be with Bill and Judy and just talk about anything and everything. The roads were not busy and the hardest part of the drive was trying to find an open restaurant to eat dinner. Luckily we came across an IHOP, and, after a few minutes of waiting, we got a table for all six of us. Dawn, Brian, Sara, Bill, Judy, and I enjoyed probably the best meal we could have had on a Christmas Day on the road. By the time we left, the place was getting pretty crowded, so we were happy that we got seated when we did.

After we arrived, we stayed in a hotel that wasn't far from where we would board the ship the next day. We got to our hotel rooms that night and tried to relax as much as we could. I had a room to myself, so I listened to my IPOD and reflected on the day.

The next morning we went to the cruise ship. Going through all the boarding process allowed us to be outside in the sunlight. I needed the brightness to take away the darkness I was attempting to climb out of. As we stood in line waiting to embark, I couldn't help but notice that everyone was with someone as I was just checking in by myself. I was thankful that Denise's family was with me, but I still felt very much alone.

We boarded the ship and our luggage was taken to be checked by security and later dropped off outside our rooms. The family and I went to find some food and get a bite. After we ate, we explored the cruise ship, which made for an enjoyable time. Denise would have liked to see this ship and go on this vacation, but those weren't the cards we were dealt.

The ship was not one of the biggest in the cruise line, but it was still plenty large to me, and I really enjoyed walking around the decks. Overall the cruise was a good escape. I stayed in a room with Sara and we had a good time cracking jokes.

The first night I woke up and went to check on her and got scared because I didn't see her. I was afraid she had fallen off the bed, but after a second I realized she just didn't sleep on the pillow (weird kid).

Spending time with Sara brightened my trip. For an eight-year-old kid, she was well ahead with her cognitive skills. She asked me questions about Denise and told me some of the reasons she missed her aunt so much. It was comforting to have someone to talk to. I had forgotten how nice it was to have someone in the room/house.

Great weather afforded an opportunity to spend a fair amount of time relaxing. We took one shore excursion on Nassau and walked around the Atlantis resort. We didn't get to visit the entire place because we would have needed to pay, but it was a beautiful resort with plenty of free sights to see.

I still found it challenging to stay still. Often when we sat by the pool, I felt I needed to be up and moving, so I got up and walked around the ship. Many times my little roommate joined me and we just strolled and talked. Sara and I were great buddies on the trip. In the afternoons somehow we always seemed to find our way to the free ice cream; it was the oddest thing.

Dinners were sumptuous and the food was as delicious as it usually is on a cruise ship. Often in the evening, I would go around the walking deck and listen to my IPOD. I liked to see people but I've never been much of a casino guy. Because I don't enjoy being around too much smoke, I usually stayed away from a lot of the evening activities. Also, even though I was on a cruise, I still hadn't been able to sleep well. I tried to keep to my routine of going to bed early so I could get as much rest as I needed.

Ever since the first night of Denise's passing, I had written to her. The cruise was not going to break that habit. I usually returned to the room early to start my writing/journaling. The cruise wasn't one of the longer cruises, so after about the second night I commented in my writing that I was having a great time but knew that after only a couple more nights I would have to head back to the empty house and the reality of my situation. As wonderful as the cruise was, I recognized the challenges I would face once it ended.

The family always seemed to have a more joyful time when we were together, and the cruise was no different. The hardest part of the day was morning. Usually I'm a big fan of breakfast, but, because we rose early there weren't many people at breakfast or at least far less than at lunch and dinner. Normally I would prefer fewer people, but the place where we ate always played music, which was much more noticeable without a crowd. Many of the songs were the melody-driven, soft tunes that really affected me. The family could tell when a song evoked my emotions even though I tried to cover it up. Twice as I heard a Jason Mraz song, I clearly couldn't hide my feelings. I ended up excusing myself at least once and went into the hallway, where there was no music, for a minute or two before returning to my food and trying to enjoy the rest of the meal.

I wasn't looking forward to the trip home but knew it was coming. We were able to disembark fairly early. We got to our cars and headed out in good timing. The plan was to drive the whole way back to our respective houses.

The thought of getting back to reality weighed heavily on me. The sad truth was that I considered what once was our home was now nothing more than shelter.

Even while on the cruise having a good time, the transition back to the emptiness of my life crept into my mind. As it turned out, the drive lasted about seven hours, and, after such a long day on the road, the feeling of just wanting to get home trumped my sadness. I was surprised at how well I handled the situation, but I knew it had more to do with the long day driving than the empty rooms.

Back in town and back to the reality, I only had a couple days before I would return to the structure of school. I also would be re-introduced to my paperwork and would start to carry more of the burden of my job with all the meetings and everything that comes with being a special education teacher.

I used those few days to clean the house. I put away all the stuff from the cruise, washed all my dress clothes, tidied the rooms, and spent a few mornings going to the gym.

On New Year's Day, I told Denise's family that I would go bowling if they would be interested in joining and sure enough they all came out. We continued our tradition of bowling on New Year's Day. It wasn't the same without Denise, but we unfortunately would have to get used to that feeling. After our outing, the rest of the family planned to go out to eat, but I decided to pass. Instead I wanted to continue the other tradition Denise and I had of eating Chinese food for lunch. I picked up takeout, took it home, and ate it by myself with my earbuds in.

I prepared everything for the first day of school. As much as I enjoyed parts of my time off, I was very much ready to get back to work and resume the routine I so desperately needed.

I realized the next hurdle to cross was going to be another difficult one. The family and I had decided that in January we would start to clean out the house, take care of all of Denise's clothes, and attempt to figure out what best to do with the nursery. This was going to be extremely difficult and much more so after a conflict between Bill, Judy, and myself before Christmas. Luckily, we were able to handle our frustration during Christmas and on the cruise; however, the main element of the conflict centered on the cleaning up of Denise's clothing.

Making these difficult decisions after a love-one's loss is something no family should have to do, but we just added this to the ever-growing pile of "things we shouldn't have to do."

I made it through the Christmas vacation, experiencing some enjoyable highs and some depressing lows. I managed to get through two of the hardest months, and, although I continued to progress, there was still an uphill climb waiting for me.

Chapter 7

Letting Go of Her Things

After Christmas, with school back in session and more structure returning in my life, I faced some difficult tasks. Some of the decisions I made prior to Christmas meant this part of Denise's death would be harder on the family.

Before Denise's family and I went on our cruise, when Mom was with me, I asked her to put some of the clothes from Denise's bedroom drawer in bags so that Judy or Dawn could decide what they wanted to do with those belongings. Early in the process, I told the family I planned to wait until after Christmas to sort through her belongings. Actually I wanted them to know that I wasn't going to touch the nursery or Denise's closet.

One evening before Christmas and the cruise while eating pizza with Bill and Judy, I mentioned that they were more than welcome to come over to look at Denise's clothes in the bags. So many of her things needed to be addressed that I needed to take the process in stages. As I cleaned out one area in a weekend, whichever parent was with me during that time helped. With my ADHD still in high gear, I had to take on one project and try to get as much accomplished as I could. Some weekends I worked on the bathroom and other weekends I started part of the office. But I hadn't managed to face touching her closet or the nursery.

After I mentioned to Bill and Judy about the drawer, I thought everything was fine. I didn't think anything of it and assumed they wanted to approach the job in stages too. As I cleaned out an area, I put piles downstairs so Bill and Judy could look at those things if they wanted while I was at work.

The next day after mentioning how mom and I cleaned out her drawer, I got a call from Bill that didn't go very well. He calmly told me that Judy really had a hard time with the fact that I would try to clean out some of Denise's things without them. He said that I had already told them I wasn't going to touch her things until after Christmas. I was shocked by this comment, but I could see his point. I did say I would wait, but I tried to explain that my statements had more to do with the big rooms like the nursery and closet.

My actions really bothered Judy, and Bill was letting me know. I tried as calmly as I could to diffuse the situation and thought I was handling myself as well as I could. I explained how difficult it had been living in the house for months with the constant reminder that the woman I loved, who owned all these things, was no longer there. They didn't have to be surrounded by all these ever-present souvenirs of a life that would never be.

As Bill talked to me, I grew more frustrated and tried to end the conversation before I blew up. I tried with every ounce of my energy to get us to end our conversation. Sadly, Bill was not understanding what I was doing, and it reached a point where I lost my cool.

I have always prided myself on my ability to act respectfully and responsibility. If things made me mad, I usually walked away until emotions settled and I was able to move on. But this time my attempts to end the conversation didn't work. I lost it. I yelled, cussed, and unloaded the sad truth that I had to live in the house and that, if I chose to do one aspect of the cleaning up, I should be able to.

I felt so angry. Two months of bottling my anger over what happened to my wife and unborn children led to an explosion of feeling. I tried desperately to end the conversation and when it didn't I was very ready to yell obscenities.

I don't think Bill had ever seen or heard me act like that; very few actually have. Bill said he didn't realize I felt that way, and I said some choice words back to him. I am not proud of how I acted. I tried frantically to keep myself together and I failed.

In dealing with this kind of tragedy and its aftermath, I wanted with all of my heart to keep the family together. To our credit we were doing far better than I could have expected. I was disappointed in how the phone call went and upset that I wasn't able to end it before I yelled at Bill. I was most frustrated with how I had reacted. Looking back, there are people with whom I could and should have been angry, but Bill was not one of them. We were all in a lot of pain already, and having this phone conversation before Christmas brought even more upset to an already distressing time. The fact that we were going to travel together for the cruise forced us all to move through our feelings. We did as well as we could and things calmed down between us before the cruise and after the holiday.

I still felt disappointed about how everything was handled, mostly my part in the family drama, and we hadn't even gotten to the hardest part yet. After Bill and I talked, Mom and I put the clothes back in the drawer, and I didn't touch anything else until Dawn and Judy had the time to come over to help clean. I still found it challenging to live in a house surrounded by her things, but I was able to manage.

In January I had to confront a challenging project. I knew there were a number of things of Denise's I wanted to keep. I spent a great deal of time and effort on my own going through the artifacts in Denise's office closet. That was where we kept her scrapbooking materials, her scrapbooks, pictures, and many of her childhood keepsakes. One weekend I decided to pull everything out and put it in the loft to sort. Sadness overwhelmed me as I went through those mementos of her life.

I saw so many beautiful pictures she had taken and things she had made. They were all so precious, those tokens of a life cut far too short. I cried like a baby. I vowed that I would go through everything. I made piles beyond piles—one for things I wanted to keep, another for her family to go through, others for items that were given to her by her closest friends.

That weekend tested my ability to focus on the task amidst so much emotion. I had to take it all in stages because I would start crying uncontrollably and have to take a break. To give myself an opportunity for release and a break from this emotional journey, I lined up calls with friends. I spoke to people I hadn't seen since college or high school. I talked to a friend with whom I had a rocky past who reached out me in my time of grief.

I worked carefully to make sure I went through all her things the correct way. As I looked through her childhood pictures and photos from her high school dances, I felt as if my heart were breaking all over again. She wore that dazzling smile in her high school formal dance picture. As I held that photo in my hands, the thought passed through my mind that our children would never experience a moment like this one their mother had.

Between the number of things to sort and the need for breaks, I realized I wasn't going to be able to finish this job in just one weekend. Luckily, I got some unexpected help. A snowstorm arrived and school was cancelled for a couple days. I would have some time to finish the project the way it should be done.

I couldn't imagine keeping all the beautiful photos littered throughout the loft. Locking myself in for two days was hard, but it was something that needed to be done. Returning to the routines of school after the tough weekend would have been therapeutic, but I needed to complete this task. Going through so many photos and mementos was traumatic, but those two extra days away from school allowed me to finish.

My good friend Ms. Davenport reached out to see how I was doing. She understood my need for structure and that being home alone for more than a weekend was tough on me. She offered to come over and we went for a walk, which helped get my thoughts and feelings out.

Being cooped up with all those memories of my beautiful wife and the sadness I felt made for a really emotional couple of days, and we hadn't even started the nursery or closet.

Rarely are there positives to school being cancelled. Since I teach in a year-round school, there are no make-up days to add to the end of the term. That means we get to do a half day of school on Saturday. Normally I hate Saturday make-ups. By the time you get home, you're tired and have only a day and a half to complete all the weekend chores you usually have two days to do. But this make-up Saturday would be good because it was going to be on the day that Dawn and Judy cleaned out Denise's closet. Me not being there was beneficial for all of us because of the unfortunate events that unfolded before Christmas. Some awkwardness remained when we were around each other, and I wanted them to be able to clear her belongings without experiencing that.

Denise was a wonderful person who was always thinking of others, but she loved to indulge in fashion and clothes. Our new house had offered her a massive closet that she quickly filled to overflowing.

Dawn and Judy came over after I had gone to school and began going through all of Denise's clothes. This seemed to be the best way to let them do what they felt they had the right to do. Although Bill and I weren't getting along perfectly, we were at least on speaking terms and could be in a room together.

As I had done with her keepsakes, Dawn and Judy sorted her clothing into a number of piles. A number of clothes were brand new and still held their price tag. I have to give Dawn and Judy credit because by the time I got home they had done a fabulous job of cleaning everything out and knew what piles they would be keeping, which they thought they could take to a consignment store, and what they would donate to the local Goodwill.

By the time I arrived home, the closet looked completely different, much sadder. It reflected what my life was at that moment. Dawn and Judy did a great job with the first part of their tough task. I was glad I didn't get in their way and that they were able to do it for their own grieving process.

That evening while listening to my iPod and brushing my teeth, I walked into the closet. It just felt weird. After I finished brushing my teeth, I turned off my iPod, took my earbuds out, and just lay in the now-empty closest and cried like a baby. Her closet looked so different, so wrong. That Saturday morning the closet brimmed with every color you could imagine and was filled with everything you could need. The only color remaining was that of the paint on the walls.

I never realized how much room the closet had and never wanted to find out. The closet was empty to match my heart. As tough as it was for me, I'm sure Dawn and Judy had a much more difficult time going through it all.

With one of the big projects pretty much completed, next came the job that brought home the painful truth that more than one person died in this tragedy. Denise and I were so ready for our twins and the nursery reflected that. That room was filled with the preparations we had made together. A place meant for happiness now held only sadness. There were two cribs, a dresser, a bookshelf, shelves on the wall, two car seats, two more car bases, a swinger, and the closet was literally filled with baby clothes, diapers, and diaper rash cream. Nothing was missing except the two little ones who were meant to live there. It was all wrong and it was my reality.

Never having been around babies, I had no idea what to do with those many items in the nursery. Again I let Dawn and Judy take the reins because I recognized how important it was to them and that I wouldn't know what do with everything. I was at the house that day and went into the room to check on them from time to time. The three of us shed many tears, but they handled the situation as well as anyone could have. No one should have to do what they did that day.

After three different baby showers, there were countless new things. Denise was so well organized that many of the baby clothes were already washed, folded, placed in the dresser and ready to be used. We had been thrilled about having a boy and a girl, and that room was a reflection of our joy. We had almost everything we could want in a nursery and two of almost everything. My heart ached remembering the happiness we shared preparing that room for our little ones.

As I worked on my own clearing and cleaning throughout the house, Dawn and Judy took care of the nursery. I was proud of how well they did, and, by the end of the day, like the closet, the nursery looked both better and worse. There were a couple odds and ends that I could take care of, but all the books and clothes were put away.

Everything was different now. The room still looked like a nursery since I would be taking care of the cribs, and the rocker was still in the corner. The room was gray and white and completely disheartening. Dawn and Judy did an amazing job in a heart-crushing situation, and I could never thank them enough for not making me do this job.

Dawn and Judy decided to find good homes for a lot of the things in the nursery, so many were donated to places that would need and use baby supplies. I gave some of the diapers to a friend who was about to have a second child. We put a few of the favorite baby shirts to the side as I wanted to keep them. We took some items to the consignment store; Dawn and Judy had a good idea about the money from those going to the memorial fund.

After Dawn and Judy left, the room was bare and closer to transferring from a nursery to a guest bedroom. There were still some things that still needed to be done, but it already looked much different from how it had 24 hours earlier.

About a month later my father came for a lengthy stay. He didn't want to come until Dawn and Judy had time to complete this task that helped with their grieving process. Dad and I planned to work on a number of projects, the biggest one being taxes. Because Denise was a pro at using TurboTax, I hadn't done my taxes since I met her.

I asked Dad to finish clearing the nursery as well. The first thing he did was move the rocker into the loft. It was a really nice rocker and I wanted to keep it, but, as long as it remained in what had been the nursery, I wouldn't be able to see it without imagining Denise sitting there holding the twins. The next thing Dad was kind enough to do was to take care of the cribs. With the help of the instructions, he did a really good job of taking apart the gray crib and putting it in the closet. We didn't know what we would do with it, but, after I told one of my friends, she said she would give me money for it if and when she and her husband had another child. I told her I would keep the crib for them until she and her husband could put it to proper use.

Denise loved babies. She was great with them and loved seeing newborns. She would have wanted the crib to find a new home, so I told my friend I wouldn't take any money for it.

"When the time comes," I said, "if you feel obliged to give something, you can write a check to Denise's fund."

Dad arranged the crib against the closet wall, keeping it out of sight to visitors. We talked about transforming the other crib into a twin bed. When Denise and I were researching which beds to buy, I was adamant about getting one that the kids could use until they left for college. Therefore, we had connections for both cribs to turn them into beds when the babies became older. Dad carefully dismantled the white crib and made it into an actual bed. The room was getting closer to no longer resembling a nursery.

Dad kindly bought a box spring and a mattress and scheduled their delivery. I deeply appreciated Dad's help with all the odds and ends that needed to be taken care of around the house. With his kindness and support, I could let go of the fear of exhausting myself with errands on weekends or having to take time away from the structure of school.

With the new bed, the room looked much less sad and a lot less intimidating to go in. Dad and I talked about what we were going to do with the dresser. While it was well-made and nice looking, the gray dresser matched the crib that was stored in the closet. It was clearly a piece of furniture meant to house baby clothes.

I came up with the idea of moving it into the downstairs guest bedroom because it would match the colors that Denise had chosen for that room. Dad and I really tried to find a way to lessen the weight of it but were unable to take the drawers out of it. Still, one way or another we were going to have to move the dresser.

I had asked my neighbor Adam if he would mind coming over to give it a look and see if he could find a way to remove the drawers. Because he is a wonderful neighbor and friend, he came to help but couldn't find a solution either to lessening the weight.

He turned to me and asked, "Do you think we can take it downstairs without removing the drawers?"

I go to the gym, but that doesn't make me strong. Dad and I are both skinny; lifting weights makes us look like we are strong, but clearly that has more to do with our thin body type rather than how much we can lift. I told Adam that I wouldn't be able to carry the bulk of it, but he acted like he thought he could take the bottom position going down the stairs.

I felt it was worth a try and, sure enough, Hercules (Adam) was amazing. He pretty much picked it up by himself, and I did my best to keep up with him. Adam was able to get it all the way downstairs and into the guest bedroom without even a scratch on the dresser or the walls. It was very impressive. Both Dad and I complimented him on his strength as well as his helpfulness. Adam was happy to assist, and we assured him that the next time we needed some muscle we would call him.

The dresser was the last item that belonged to the nursery. With it gone and the box spring and mattress delivered, the room felt different, not better, just different. Before everything was taken apart, I took a final picture of the room to remind me how it once looked when we lived in joyful anticipation

---

of the birth of our babies. We had it all then. In the end I had nothing.

The house was slowly transforming from Denise's home to my residence. I knew I had to make it my own, but, of the two of us, Denise was the interior decorator. I kept everything as it was and even added some pictures of Denise and me up to the walls.

I'm proud of how well the entire family came together to do this. I still am disappointed in myself for how I handled the initial issue of talking to Bill on the phone, but there is a reason many families have conflicts after the death of a loved one. We were no longer each other's best friends and things would never be the same. Nevertheless, we united as a family when faced with a challenge as monumental as cleaning out that nursery and Denise's closet.

The house will never be what it should have been, but this was the world we now lived in. At least as we proceeded through our grieving. There were still things that needed to be done; we could still function as a family, and one that was somehow surviving.

Chapter 8

Being in Public

As the house was becoming my home, I struggled with a lot of internal issues. The psychological ramifications of transitioning from such shared love and excitement to complete emptiness and sadness were excruciating. Sadly, though, I had no say in this life and had to suffer through the only existence I would get.

I continued to do what needed to be done. Before Christmas I had decided that I would attempt to move back into our bedroom, which was difficult for a number of reasons. The bedroom was the place at the start of the darkness, where Denise's life had ended. I hadn't slept in that bed for a while. But this was another obstacle I had to face.

One thing that eased my transition to the bedroom was the use of a heavy air freshener. For a while I couldn't go into the bedroom without smelling death in the air. A musty odor permeated the space. That scent will haunt me for the rest of my life. I soon realized that to be able to go into the bedroom without horrific images rising into my consciousness, I had to alter the smell of the room. I will forever connect that smell to the images imprinted on my psyche that fateful morning, so I will probably always need an air freshener in that space.

With the elimination of the odor and the images it conjured into my mind, I could think about moving back into the bedroom. It was not something I wanted to do, but I felt Denise would have wanted me to. A couple of days before I planned to move back into the room, I just lay on the bed and watched the TV to get my head where it needed to be with the upcoming transition.

I felt nervous on that first night, but it didn't turn out to be that bad. Being on sleep meds apparently make transitions like this much easier to cope with. I remained a little uneasy for a while, but the medication did its work, and I was able to make it through the night. Sleep was still pretty tough for me as I continued to deal with a lot of anger and sadness. I worried about waking up in the middle of the night, needing to go to the bathroom, and being unable to fall back asleep.

I ate dinner early in hopes of getting all the "waste" out of my system before I tried to fall asleep. On those occasions when I still couldn't make it through the night, it was nice to just put on the TV; then I could still try to relax my body.

Work continued to be a good distraction for me and a great way to gain the structure I so desperately needed. For eight hours of my day, I had something that required my attention and focus. Then I only had to worry about filling 3.5 hours before I started my evening routines to get ready for bed.

My students gave me so much support through this time. Their consistent smiles and help eased my days and brought some comfort in a world that wasn't meant for my happiness.

My weekends continued to follow the same routines, and church was the main place where I cried. I reserved most of my Sunday mornings for Denise. Sundays would be my time to cry at her niche. I tried not to cry too much during the service but instead held my tears until I sat in front of her niche. Afterward I came home and watched the film of the viewing that Dawn and Brian made and cried some more.

Weeping may be viewed as something weak people do. But I was becoming aware of the emotional release I got from crying. It takes strength to be willing to let those feelings flow out.

I had to take water with me to church on Sunday mornings. Otherwise all the crying could leave me dehydrated and much more prone to get headaches by the afternoon.

With February arriving, I knew I had a couple things coming up that were going to be difficult. I had made it through Thanksgiving and Christmas, but the "year of firsts" kept coming, and before too long I had to get through Valentine's Day.

The other upcoming issue was attempting to prepare our tax returns. Even before Denise and I were officially together, she had done my taxes. This year's taxes were going to be difficult for a number of reasons. However, with the house in better shape than it was last year and my Dad fully retired, he agreed to spend a good deal of time with me to help with doing taxes as well as a long list of other tasks.

Not everyone who goes through something like this has the flexibility to have family members visit and help them with a lot of the issues that arise from tragedies on this level. I was lucky to have a great deal of support. My Dad could help with many of these things so I didn't have to lose the structure of school. Dad found a woman who could file our taxes, and she did a wonderful job. His support in working on the nursery and countless other projects meant the world to me.

After Denise's passing, I was left with two cars. I didn't need both of them, but I wasn't ready to get rid of one yet. There was a lot of discussion about which car I should sell. Since our new Explorer was less than a year into the three-year lease and I liked sitting high in the SUV more than getting down into the Ford Fusion, I decided to sell the Fusion.

Dad and I had some idea about how much it would sell for because of some paperwork we had to give the estate lawyer. One Saturday, Dad followed me into Raleigh, and we were able to sell the Fusion. We got a bit less than we wanted, but it was more something that needed to be done. In the moment of Denise's passing, I had no notion of what would follow. Although the sadness remained, the countless jobs needed to be completed.

With Dad in town, I was able to come home to someone at the house. He and I often took walks after school to just talk. I enjoyed hearing about what he did each day and craved conversation by the end of school. It felt much better coming home to see Dad than it did when the house was empty.

I also continued to engage in more conversation on my Sunday walks with a support person named Mr. Bob (more on him later). Mr. Bob and I talked a lot about how he felt I was progressing, how things were holding up at school, movies we saw, and North Carolina State basketball. I was still working on trying to set up the 5K for Denise's fund, and Bob and I explored places where I might hold a possible race.

As I progressed through my pain, my Uncle Mike's health continued to be challenging for him. He hadn't been well before Denise's passing, but I didn't realize until I saw him how much he was suffering. When he came for the funeral, his health challenges were evident. Some days Mike wouldn't want to talk by phone, but I tried to reach out to him. Dad had stopped by the post office one afternoon and had bought some postcards. I sent Mike a postcard every couple of days. My uncle had always been a wonderful guy, and it made me feel good that, even in my sadness, I could do something kind for him. I had read in my grief books that people in pain such as mine sometimes feel better when they help others. Letting Mike know I was thinking of him definitely made me feel good. I only wished his health would improve.

I expected Valentine's Day to be difficult. I had bought Denise a Valentine's Day card and after work I drove to the church, sat by her niche, and talked to her. I read her what I wrote and cried. Valentine's Day is meant to be about love, not the sadness I was feeling. I can't imagine I will ever have a worse Valentine's Day than I did that year. However, after I left the church and went home to see and talk to Dad, I felt less alone and anguished.

While I usually came straight home after work, I will say there were some thoughtful friends who reached out and tried to get me to move outside my comfort zone on occasion. I used to be a social person, but I had loved staying at home with Denise on Friday and Saturday nights. We rarely went out and instead enjoyed the comfort of our love. Going out less than most meant being able to save for our various expenses.

Now that I was essentially living by myself, I felt torn about going places. I had continued going to church, which entailed being in public to a degree. However, I didn't really talk to anyone. I didn't have anything to say and often spent my time during the music portion of the service trying not to cry. The pastors were kind to me but understood that I didn't say much and that most of my focus was visiting the niche to be close to the only part of Denise that was left.

The other public place I went weekly was the supermarket. Every Friday night whenever my parents weren't in town I shopped for groceries. My parents took over this responsibility when they were in town. Grocery shopping was something Denise and I both loved and hated. We enjoyed the time together but weren't big fans of the shopping experience itself; we did it on Friday evening to get it behind us and have the rest of the weekend free.

The first time I went to the supermarket by myself I almost cried. I did my best to hold my emotions in check. Even after the first visit, I still felt sadness threaten to overtake me on this trips when I walked by a certain food that Denise loved or saw something that reminded me of her. Just performing the task that we usually shared together left me feeling the strain of missing her. While I did not enjoy these necessary shopping trips, making the effort was a step in the right direction. It took some time for me to be able to do it without getting emotional.

There were other occasions in public that presented profound challenges for me. The moment I will never forget was the morning I went to get my blood drawn, the same terrible day I walked into Denise's OB/GYN to pick up her medical records.

My doctor, who was and is a wonderful representative of the medical community, had been worried about my health from the moment she saw that the medical examiner's office asked for Denise's records. I had met my doctor through Denise, who had wonderful things to say about her. Once Denise and I were together, her doctor agreed to take me on as a patient as well.

I think our doctor was heartbroken to learn of Denise's passing. Soon after she heard of the news, she reached out to me to try to touch base about how I was doing and, honestly, to show me she cared deeply for Denise. She is definitely a wonderful lady.

When I spoke with her, my doctor said it would be a good idea for me to do a check-up and maybe get some blood drawn. I agreed and went in during my Christmas break to have it done. Since I was going to be next door to Denise's OB/GYN, I figured I would call and ask for her records. They let me know what forms I would need to bring and told me that they would make a copy of the records for me to pick up.

That morning I woke up and immediately drove over to get my blood taken. I wasn't able to eat anything but kept a banana in the car to have as soon as I got my blood drawn. I planned to go to the Chick-Fil-A across the street afterward and get some food before stopping in at the OB/GYN office.

Getting blood drawn was no big deal to me since I did it quite frequently as a child. As soon as I was finished, I ate my banana and went to Chick-Fil-A for breakfast. The smart move would have been to visit the drive-through and eat in my car. However, I knew I needed to see how I would handle myself. I headed inside, ordered my food, and sat down.

Sitting in a booth by yourself is awkward, but doing it with my current mental state was horrible. I kept having to look out the window so the other customers couldn't see the tears in my eyes. I'm sure I cried on my breakfast and then ate the tears. It was a tough moment and one that I will never forget for the rest of my life.

I hated what I had become. I used to be the happy guy who enjoyed sitting places and people watching. Now I was the guy who couldn't function in public and stared out the window to avoid affecting the other customers. It was a tough morning.

I was able to get myself together after I ate, probably the fastest breakfast meal ever, and made it over to the OB/GYN office. I got her medical records, asked a question about a refund check I received, and then spent the next 20 minutes in my car looking over her file. If that morning taught me anything, it was that I was still not able to function in public if I wasn't able to move around.

There were other issues I was facing and realizing about myself. I was able to function well at school, but a large part of that had to do with the fact that I was active at work. It also helped that my students were wonderful kids and brought out the best in me during those tough months. However, I didn't talk much since I was no longer "drying up the well" before the kids came into my class in the morning, and I had little to say after the students left at the end of the day.

Every year one of our big school fundraisers was an event called "O'Holly Night," a title that plays off the town and school name of Holly Springs. During this fundraiser there is a blind drawing for baskets that each teacher's class put together centered around a particular theme. Denise would always come over to my school for the event. She would pick up Subway for the two of us; then we would eat in my room before going to the library to look at all the baskets before it got too crowded. Denise used to love picking which baskets we would try to win and selecting how many tickets we put into which baskets. You should have seen the expression on her face the year we won the "Let the Restaurants Do the Cooking" basket. It contained lots of restaurant gift cards and two cards for a free meal every month at Noodles & Company for a year.

Now I was caught in this weird place, being there without Denise. I wanted to support the school but knew I wasn't in the right mood to see all those happy families. I decided to put in all my tickets and leave without talking to anyone. I drove home to the empty house.

That evening as I was constructing a Lego set, I heard I had won a basket. I feel bad saying this, but I was deeply saddened by winning a basket. I wished I hadn't won the barbeque basket (with charcoal grill). My first reaction when I saw the text message that I had won was sadness, because this was a moment I deeply wanted to share with Denise.

I felt like I didn't want good things to happen to me because I didn't have anyone with whom I could share these moments. I was relieved that I didn't stay for the event because people would have been happy for me winning the basket, and I wouldn't have known how to handle my sadness and emptiness in the moment.

I was starting to understand my view of spending time in public. For a time around Christmas, I held some hope about the possibility of finding a degree of normalcy at public events. One day at school, I was eating lunch in my classroom as always while listening to ESPN radio. One of the other few male teachers came in. He asked if I would come with the 4th grade team for dinner after school. In the moment I thought that I could manage that and told him I'd like to. However, after a little time passed, I realized I just couldn't bring myself to go with them. Looking back on it, I probably should have made an attempt. These friends would have been the best people to spend some time with. But I was battling with this internal issue of how to be honest with people but also not ruin their fun. I didn't want to be fake and pretend that everything was okay when clearly it wasn't. At the same time, I didn't want to hold anyone back from having a good time.

I ended up telling this teacher that I just couldn't do it. I think he understood. I let him know that it meant a lot to me that he asked. I think the moral to this part of the story is that often people don't ask questions if they feel they already know the answer. However, this time I was so glad that he invited me to join them because it showed that he cared. Even though we know what the answer will be, sometimes just asking the question is a kind gesture. I will forever remember that he went out of his way for me and was understanding when I went back on my word.

My goal at that point was simply to keep staying alive even if that meant coming home every night to waste the hours. I was living in this world and I was maintaining my own sanity. I couldn't be around others and that was okay. I didn't have much to say to people, and the more I kept to myself, the more I would probably keep myself isolated. This was the only way I felt that I could handle my situation.

I didn't know how to act in public. I had always been good around people because I was happy. Now that I was sad, empty, and depressed, I could never seem to find the right words. It was a difficult time.

In the past, one of the things that made me such a fun guy to be around was the fact that I was always happy and outgoing. The contrast to my former self made a lot of my current circumstances more challenging.

As bad as my life was, I wasn't bringing more sadness into other people's lives. Knowing that helped me feel better. I got a little bit of happiness knowing that other people were happy even if it made my life a lot sadder by contrast. I have always said that I didn't want my diluted view of the world to affect others. The sad truth is that if you live by that belief you're further isolating yourself from those who can help.

Even in those days, I could find a little comfort in simple things. I didn't need to put myself out there and pretend that life was going to end up great. One good thing I did was to accept a couple of invitations from my wonderful neighbors to play cards with them. I had explained to Adam and Tricia a number of times I wanted to be social but found it challenging to spend time in a large group of people. They helped me realize that I could find contentment and ease by playing cards with their family. I even got to laugh a little. These card games offered an escape from my life and empty house for a couple hours with people who understood that I wasn't okay.

They accepted me as I was in the moment. I was happy to find this little distraction from all the issues I had going on in my head. I wasn't ready to be *in public*, but I could manage small social situations like playing cards or talking about sports. I was grateful for their invitation and glad I accepted.

I didn't need to maintain my composure all the time. The only parts of the day I truly had to keep myself together were those hours when the kids were in my class. Other than that, I could be totally dysfunctional.

One of the advantages of being by yourself is that no one gets to see you at your worst. I had a lot of difficult times. It helped a great deal when my parents stayed with me, but those days had to end as I needed to come to terms with the emptiness that my future was going to hold. The sad truth was that I had a lot of anger and questions about how this happened. Sadly, I wasn't getting the answers I needed to help my healing.

Chapter 9

Religion

I have never been an overtly religious person. I was brought up as a Methodist and attended church regularly as a child. I have battled with religion on and off for a long time. My main concern with dogma comes down to expectations.

One of the things I like best about myself is that I can have a conversation with anyone. I have always been welcoming and accepting of almost anyone. The main reason comes from the fact that I understand how lucky I was to have the upbringing I did. I've never been really smart. I have always realized that if things didn't fall into place for me I could have ended up with a very different life. My parents did an amazing job with me as a child, and I was fortunate to be able to have the life I had as a child. Not everyone has the luxury of my upbringing, and I never took it for granted.

When I went to college, I understood that I was fortunate and really felt for others who weren't as lucky as I was. Ever since high school, I have always worked diligently. I was not gifted with book smarts, which could be both a curse and a blessing. The down side was that I dealt with a fair amount of frustration going into the education department because my ACT score wasn't up to their standards. But once I was finally able to get in, I made the grade by being persistent and tenacious. I always worked hard because I didn't have that pure smarts that others had. Because of my background, I've felt comfortable conversing with all different kinds of people. I've always understood how fortunate I was to receive the opportunities and the values I was given.

In college, I spent time with those who liked to party and those who didn't. I enjoyed hanging out with my friends at night and having a couple drinks but didn't use drugs although they were available. I often left parties early and went to bed early with plans to have breakfast with my religious friends the next day.

I always assumed and expected that my spiritual friends saw me as an open person who could talk and listen to all kinds of people. That was not the case. Often judgment arose when I interacted with those who used alcohol or drugs. I always felt that, because I didn't live other people's lives, it wasn't my place to tell them how they should act or to judge their decisions.

My views on religion were filtered through the lens of the Golden Rule: Treat others the way you would want to be treated. Often the extremely religious people I encountered didn't follow this rule as I would have expected. I believed that was what God wanted us all to do.

I probably have different views from others, and I am okay with that. We are each unique and that's a good thing. However, all of that came into question when facing the type of adversity I had to confront.

I lived a clean and healthy life and, although I had faith in God, I also believed in Karma. Overall, I believed that if I lived a caring, kind, responsible life, I would be rewarded. When Denise and I were really struggling to get pregnant, I questioned this. But when we found out that she was pregnant and that we would be having twins, a boy and a girl, my views on Karma and the rewards for a life well lived grew. I was ecstatic when we received that news. Denise and I were good people and we would create a loving family.

Everything changed after she and our unborn twins left this world. I used to pray every night for the thing we wanted most in the world, healthy babies. I would talk to God and ask Him to help us bring two healthy infants into the world. I felt that, if He gave us that, we would make this world a better place by trying our best and raising those kids with love, instilling in them the values and beliefs we shared.

Sadly, when Denise died and those babies passed with her, I went down a dark road with respect to religion. Even then, I still respected and valued some of the great aspects of religion and the people who are faithful.

The people at the church were amazing to us. They went out of their way to help Denise's family and me through the grieving process. They relieved us of one burden by allowing us to have both the viewing and the funeral on their property. As bad as it was, we were surrounded by some of the kindest people during that first week. From the police officers to the funeral home employees to the people who worked and volunteered at the church, we found kindness at every turn. They cared about us as individuals and as a grieving family. They offered every kind of aid you could want when you are going through the sadness that we experienced. On top of how compassionate they were, they also identified how much help we would need going forward. The sad truth was this was going to be our reality for a long time to come.

The church did a wonderful job of trying to find a Stephen Minister for me. Stephen Ministry is an organization that helps people when dealing with sadness or death. Our church had a couple of these volunteers, and they were kind enough to help me and match me with a man I knew as Mr. Bob.

Mr. Bob had been around the block, dealing with death personally as well as helping others during the times of a loved one's passing, and had helped a number of people before he met me. However, most of those with whom he worked weren't my age. It's a painful thing to deal with a loved one's death at such a young age. It's difficult at any age. However, my story was different in that it wasn't just a wife that I lost. This added an additional element to my sadness. I was taught early in the process not to compare my grief to others. But in truth I sometimes wished I had another person's grief and not my own. It's not a good thing to say, but, speaking honestly from my heart, I definitely had that thought.

Bob and I were together for countless hours and took many walks. The first time he came over to talk with me I explained that my brain seems to work best through movement. Bob was nice enough to agree to walk with me, and soon our Sunday afternoons together became a routine and a way to get out of the house.

Bob was wonderful to me. He really listened. We talked about anything and everything. He was a big North Carolina State fan, so we talked about college sports at length. Since we both enjoyed movies, we found ourselves conversing about films as well on those occasions when I wanted to talk about something other than Denise's passing.

Unlike a therapist, Bob and I had open dialogue and conversation. I spoke much of the time about how I was feeling, but I really liked listening to Bob converse about his life and hearing his stories. I was lucky to have Bob assigned to me; his presence was a constant comfort to me through my grief and sadness.

The hard part about our relationship was that he was attempting to support my overall wellbeing and aid me in my faith. My anger at the medical community and at God was intense at the time. Bob and I had a lot of talks about our individual views, and I'm sure that the darkness I spoke about was difficult for him to hear.

However, every week Bob spent time with me and continued to support me and bring comfort. He is someone who really cares. His kindness goes far beyond the norm. Bob had the devotion and dedication to walk and talk with me every Sunday. I was fortunate to have met such a wonderful person. Of course, I wished with all my heart that I never had met him because of the tragedy that brought our lives together. He understood that.

Bob and I spent hours talking about God's role in this tragedy. Bob and I didn't agree on everything. However, we were both willing to hear the other person's point of view and have an open discussion. He was aware that my emotions were raw and that in time things would get better. However, when you are living in the moment, you don't want to think about the future. When you exist inside the grief I had, you live in survival mode. My goal was to make it to the 23rd of every month so I could say I survived another month.

Although Bob heard me say a lot of hateful things, he didn't judge me. He recognized the value of releasing my emotions even if they were toxic. I had a lot of anger directed at two outlets: the medical community and God. I felt so much rage toward God for this profound loss.

"When I die, the first thing I'll do when I get to heaven is hug my family," I once told Bob. "The second thing I'll do is punch God right in the face."

I'm sure it wasn't the smartest thing to say, but it was a feeling I had. I knew my wife was worried about her health; Denise and I had sat in meetings with people explaining the potential issues of an at-risk pregnancy. But I put my faith in God to get her to a place where those babies were full-term. Then when she died, in my heart I felt that God had failed me and Denise and those twins. Those babies would never be able to see the world. Denise would never get to read to them or watch them grow up. I would never get to see Denise become the amazing mother I knew she would be. I felt God had taken that from us.

As Bob and I carried on an open dialogue about the role of God and whether God allowed for free will or was a micromanager, the one thing I kept coming back to was that I felt God could have prevented this. I'm sure that God doesn't like when tragedies happen, and I've read books about miracles. But for whatever reason saving Denise and those babies was not one of those miracles.

It seemed so wrong to me and I will always question God's role in what happened. My emotions were raw. I had so much anger that the only way to get away from that was to say what I felt, and Bob took everything in stride. He was a great friend. He saw a side of me that few people will ever get to know. My healing was not going as well as we all would have hoped, but at least I had people in my corner, and, apart from the family, Bob was always there for me.

The church was caring to me and the rest of the family. I continued to attend weekly because that's where the closest physical remembrance of Denise was, her niche containing the urn that held her and the children's ashes. Bill, Judy, and I went to the contemporary program at 9:30 a.m. These services began with a lot of music. While many of the songs were written to be uplifting, Bill, Judy, and I were in mourning. It is difficult to look around and see people in church smiling and believing in those positive words while the three of us suffered through this world.

My dad, who knew how challenging the experience was for me emotionally, discussed whether he thought it was worth going to church. Both my parents are religious, but Dad was coming from a place of compassion. The traditional service would probably have been a better fit for me, but there were a couple reasons I continued to go to the 9:30 program. The first was related to the hour. It was the time I walked into our bedroom and my life changed forever. I chose to honor Denise's memory by doing something she wanted us to do more, to attend church, at an hour I will always remember. I couldn't rewrite the past, but I could choose to remember her in this way. The second reason was that I have always believed that sometimes the best things to do are the hardest.

From the very beginning of this sadness, I told people that I didn't want to take the easy way out and that often the easy path is the road that doesn't get you to where you need to be. I needed to take the difficult passageway because I felt in the long run that was the best way to become the person I should be after this. As much as I tried to hold the tears in during the service, the songs that uplifted others in faith often evoked deep feelings of sorrow in me. Still, I liked the fact that I could look around the room and see people who were in the moment. Many of them smiled and appeared uplifted by those songs, understanding how great God can be. Although I couldn't feel that joy, I appreciated knowing there were people who lived the kind of life I so desperately wanted.

As hard as the church service was, the part of the morning that was equally difficult and meaningful was my time sitting outside in the columbarium by Denise's niche. My emotions became uncontrollable on many occasions as I sat there and sobbed, even drooling on myself from crying so hard. I hated what my life had become. I was 35 years old and have seen the love of my life die.

The columbarium at the church was a beautiful place. I had never heard of this kind of place prior to her death. Again, the best description is a locker for urns. One such vessel held the remains of Denise and our twins and someday will house my remains. Each spot has a marble cover with an engraving, and the niche, which is her location in the columbarium, was close to where I sat. I have spent too many hours sitting there weeping and far too few to ever imagine enough tears had been shed.

I have seen other columbariums and the one holding Denise's ashes is to me one of the more beautiful. I have visited others that were shaded by trees in dark places. Others were off to the side of the church and a couple were across the parking lot. Although all held their own kind of beauty, I felt the columbarium where Denise rests was the nicest I have seen. It feels like part of the church. I am fortunate the woman I will always love has a resting place as lovely as it can be under these sad circumstances.

Many times, churchgoers have seen me sitting there crying and having a hard time. People have offered me hugs. Others just acknowledged me, which I appreciated. The church members and staff knew I spent time there before and after the service. Once they kindly left a card for me that everyone had signed. It was such a compassionate gesture. I appreciated the fact that they would think of me with all the other people they were supporting. I felt less alone that day. Although I was there by myself much of the time, it meant a great deal to know they were thinking of me.

The church does a considerate thing at the holidays by holding a service for people who aren't in the happy spirit of Christmas. Instead of poinsettias filling the sanctuary, boxes of tissue were placed around the space. A couple reading offered some words about the holidays that were more appropriate to the audience. It was a relief to allow myself to cry. The holidays present profound challenges to some of us, and it's thoughtful when churches identify those who struggle through the season.

The church also provided a grief share class that Bill, Judy, and I attended. It lasted 15 weeks for a couple hours every week. I was the youngest person there, but there were a number of people who were in various stages of grief. It was reassuring and helpful to listen to other people talk about how they were handling their emotions. Looking back, I don't know how much I truly got out of the class, but I was glad I went. Trying to put various pieces of support in place was a step in the right direction.

One of the really amazing things that happened to me, which carried an element of religion, was something that will always stick with me. One of Denise's relatives asked if she could stop over one night to bring dinner. I told her I would be home since I was continuing to stay in the house but still valued when people took time out of their lives to come check on me.

When she showed up, she brought a nice dinner and a card for me from some of the people she knew who participated in an exercise group that had a religious component to it. The group had heard my story and decided to raise money for me. The card held their attempts to show me there were people who cared. It contained over a thousand dollars.

I really didn't know what to say. It was difficult to imagine that there were people who would try to help even though we had never met. It was an amazing gesture.

I didn't know what to do with the money at first but came to the conclusion that I would spend it on an elliptical machine. Since they were an exercise group, I thought spending it on some type of fitness equipment would always remind me of them and that there is good in this world.

I had found that exercising was a good release for me. I have always exercised and, unlike the year before Denise's passing, had spent a large amount of time running. However, my knees had started to hurt, so I quit because I didn't want to be the guy who had to ice his knees after taking the twins for a walk. I could use the elliptical, a machine that is like running but better on one's knees, before work since there was not enough time to always get to the gym before school.

I also found that when I exercised on the elliptical on Sunday mornings I seemed to do better at the niche and at church. The gym opened after church services, so this option of exercising at home gave me a chance to release before going.

The kindness of these strangers who went out of their way to be generous made me continue my belief in the religious community. These people cared regardless of whether or not they knew me.

The sad truth of the situation was it was all still so wrong in my head. I would have given anything to go back to the way things were for Denise and me. Unfortunately, that could never happen. But because of the tragedy, these people reached out to help me, and their kindness meant the world to me.

I was honored by all the support I received, but I still had to face driving home to an empty house each day and sleeping in an empty bed every night. The next morning I would wake up in that same hollow life and do the whole thing over again. I believed in the power of God and I put my faith in Him to give Denise and me the family we worked so hard for. In the end, God gave us some of the most beautiful gifts in the world, and, at the height of what was to be our greatest happiness, it all disappeared.

I don't feel that God took Denise and those babies away on purpose. However, if you believe that God can perform miracles and that He has infinite power, then you understand that He could have prevented this horrible tragedy.

I do believe with my heart that one day I will go to heaven and get to be with those twins and Denise. When that time comes, I will have some questions I would like to ask God about why He didn't intervene and why He allowed this to happen. I realize there is bad in the world, and I know tragedies occur all the time. I just wish this wouldn't have happened to us, or, if someone had to die, I wish God had taken me and let Denise have those kids on Earth. She would have been the most amazing mom, but unfortunately she will have to do that in heaven. We didn't go through all those trials of getting pregnant so she could be a mother in heaven; we went through everything so that she could be a mom here on Earth. This was a tragedy that should never have happened and one that I think God could have prevented but chose not to.

Chapter 10

More Death

As I continued to battle with my own emotions, anger, and sadness, I managed to perform well at school. The kids I taught were really good for me. Many of them had been my students for five years, and I was doing my best to prepare them for the challenges of middle school. One of the advantages of teaching special education is often you get to keep your students as long as they are in your school. Although this is not always the case, when you make good connections with your kids, being able to work with them over multiple years is wonderful.

As much as I loved my work and my students, school continued to be exhausting as well. Although I no longer needed to "drain the well," I continued to exercise daily. Still, by the weekend I relied heavily on relaxing as much as possible to get my body ready for Monday morning.

Living in a house by yourself and doing all the cooking, cleaning, and the yard work demands a great deal of energy. I've never been a guy who likes to take time off work. When Denise was alive, I took off when she was on a break, which amounted to about one week every three months. However, toward the end of the school year, I kept working. Many years I wouldn't take off any weeks between May and August because of the demands of wrapping up the year and putting in place expectations for the next year.

Since I was going through all of this emotional turmoil, I knew I needed to do a better job of trying to break up the structure of school with time off. I had planned on taking a week's vacation in March and driving to see my parents. I love my parents and spending time with them. Unintentionally, I actually took off the Thursday and Friday of the opening round of the NCAA basketball tournament or March Madness. This trip was going to be the first time I had driven a good distance by myself.

I had traveled for the Christmas cruise with Bill and Judy, which made that an easier excursion. This trip was going to be a little tougher because I was alone in the car. I set up all my podcasts and enjoyed listening to them on the drive. I knew at some point I would have to stop for lunch, and I wasn't sure how that would go. Eventually I pulled in at a Subway to use up a gift card.

I did pretty well until I sat down. Eating by myself was still challenging. I felt the tears coming, so I ate as quickly as I could, finished my sandwich, and jumped back into my car. I was sad that I still wasn't able to eat without the fear of crying in public but glad I was at least trying to put myself in public, even if I still wasn't myself.

After lunch the rest of the trip went well. As soon as I got to my parents, I was greeted by Wags, their neurotic and hyper dog. I brought my stuff into the house and then hung out by the TV, watching the basketball games and spending time with my parents. My parents and I have a great relationship. That hasn't always been true, but, since about the time I went to college, we have gotten along really well.

The week was something that I needed very much. We spent the week taking Wags for walks, watching a whole lot of college basketball, taking little trips to town, and playing card games. It was a really great escape. My parents and I were always doing something, which seemed to help a great deal with keeping my mind off the sadness. I was very fortunate to be able to get a busy and enjoyable week away from school, and one that brought me no stress.

As the week came to an end, I was not looking forward to returning home. I easily got used to being in a home with people, laughter, and conversation. I knew what I had in front of me, returning to an empty house. Going back home was difficult, but then again it shouldn't have been easy. I stopped on the way home and bought groceries. By the time I arrived, I began preparing for getting back into the swing of things the next day with work. It was a wonderful trip but now I needed to come back to reality, even though it wasn't the reality I wanted.

The transition back to school actually was pretty good. I seemed to very quickly get reacclimated to the structure, routine, and procedures of school, and I think the kids were happy to have me back. I was about to enter one of the busier times in my schedule. For every 5th grader for whom I was the "case manager" (paperwork person), we conducted a transition meeting to discuss how we wanted them to best be served in middle school. Of all the meetings I have at school, and there are a lot of them, these were always my favorites. The reason I enjoyed them so much was that we focused only on what was important. Our conversation was centered on a couple key issues. Many of the other meetings I held dealt primarily with paperwork; we sometimes lost our focus on the important issues because there was so much else to cover.

Soon after my trip, I found myself working at a hectic pace with the preparations, holding the meeting, and the post-work of all the transition meetings for my 5th graders. It was good to be as busy as I was coming back to work.

Toward the end of March, the best man from my wedding, Tim, took time away from his family to come from Ohio and spend a weekend with me. Tim is always fun to be around. I had known him for years; he was my summer boss before I met Denise. Since I first started working in a traditional school, I had my summers off, so I would go back to the Columbus Zoo and Aquarium and help with their summer camp program. Back then I was a 27-year-old still living in my parent's basement, a fact that Tim never let me forget. He had been a great boss and a true friend. Our friendship continued over the years, and he has always been a good man.

It was really cool having someone at the house, making me laugh, even if it was only for a weekend. We watched some Netflix comedy specials and went to see a movie at the local theater. I showed him Denise's resting place, and he sat there with me as I cried. The sad part about Tim's visit is it will always be remembered as the time I found out about my Uncle Mike.

Uncle Mike continued to struggle with his health even with people helping him. I called and talked to him once a week, and I still tried to write him a postcard every other day. Helping others seemed to ease a little of the pain I felt. While Tim was visiting me, I was scanning Facebook and saw a post about how Mike had gone missing. I hadn't heard anything about this and figured I needed to call my parents.

I got in touch with Dad who informed me of the sad news. The family had hired someone to assist Mike early in the mornings. One morning when this person arrived, he wasn't home. Mike had gone missing and his truck had been found by one of the nearby lakes. My Dad felt bad that I found out from Facebook, but I told him that I understood. I probably would have chosen not to tell me if I had been in his shoes.

The fact was that Mike was missing, but, until he showed up or at least his body appeared, not much could be done.

After I hung up the phone, my first reaction was being scared for Mike. I hoped he was found quickly because the longer he went without his medication the less chance there was that this situation would end well. The call left me feeling frightened and sad. There was little I could do beyond hoping for the best and being prepared for the worst.

The rest of Tim's trip went as well as could be expected, and we enjoyed each other's company. I told Tim to thank his wife for letting me borrow him for a couple days as it was probably one of the few times I looked forward to coming home for a weekend. Tim returned home safely, and I turned my focus back to school as I hoped that Mike was all right.

The next day at school I felt strange. I kept searching the internet for more information about Mike. At the time they didn't appear to have any new leads. Over the next couple of days, the reality of the situation sank in, and I worried about how I would handle the news if Mike were deceased. I hoped he would be found living, but, with each day that went by, the likelihood of that became smaller.

Dad and I talked about the situation every couple of days. One of my big concerns was that I hoped that he didn't hurt anyone in his current state. Mike was an amazingly gentle soul, but with his mental health issues and lack of medication while missing, I was worried about what the outcome was going to be.

A couple of days later the news came out that Mike had been found and had passed away. I was scared how I was going to handle the situation, but, when the news finally came out, I was actually a little relieved. I would have much preferred that Mike was able to get the help he desperately needed. But, most importantly, I was just thankful that Mike wasn't in any more pain. He had been in distress for a while, and I really didn't realize how much he had been dealing with until I saw him when he came for Denise's funeral. After that, he had a hard time even eating. I was sad about Mike no longer being with us, but I found great comfort in the fact that he was no longer in the pain that he had carried with him for so long.

With Mike's passing, I knew he was in heaven with Denise and the twins. After so much grief, I had to make sure I got my head back to where it was previously. Two difficult milestones were quickly approaching.

The first was my birthday. I had no idea how in the world I was going to celebrate my 35th birthday, but I knew there was only one person I wanted to be close to on that day. Denise was beautiful; one of the characteristics I miss most about her was when she rolled her eyes at one of my jokes. While I was in college, I had purchased an amazing baby blue three piece suit that I always kidded I was going to wear for Denise. She was not a fan of it and made many jokes about it. She even offered to burn it for me. I never got to wear that suit for her, so I figured it was the only thing I could do on my birthday under the circumstances.

In addition to the quality of this outfit, Denise wasn't enthusiastic about a couple of bolo ties I purchased a couple months before her passing. We were driving to get some food after Denise had her haircut when she mistakenly remarked that there was a Western store on the other side of the restaurant. I was delighted by that and told her I was going over to see if they had any bolo ties. Sure enough, the store carried them. Denise rolled her eyes in a big way when I showed her my purchase and told her how inexpensive they were.

Birthdays are times of celebration, and there wasn't much for me to celebrate that year. I didn't even want my birthday to arrive. It was just another sad occasion during "the year of firsts." At school, I wanted to treat it like any other day. I planned to spend my evening at her niche. I had asked the secretary not to mention that it was my birthday, and, after I told her why, she kindly agreed to my request. However, Facebook struck again. A number of people wished me a happy birthday even though there was no happy in the birthday that year.

After school, I picked up a to-go sushi roll and went home. I put on my best outfit, the suit and bolo tie, and went and sat by Denise's niche while I ate. It will probably always be the worst birthday I will ever have. The sad truth is it also will be one I will never forget. I hated the day. I hated what it stood for. But, sadly, it was just another thing I hated in the world.

The second milestone that I was about to encounter was going to be the six-month anniversary of Denise's passing. For the longest time I didn't know what to do but realized it was going to be a painful day. I had spoken to my good friend Derek about possibly driving up to his place in Baltimore to just get away during that time. He and his wife were more than accommodating and welcomed me into their house for five evenings.

Denise and I had spent a lot of time with Derek and Gena over the years. We went to East Carolina University football games, Derek and I each passed out in weird places (restaurant bathroom floors and house toilets), and, after Derek and Gena moved to Baltimore, we always talked about going to visit them. We never found the time to drive up together before Denise's passing.

The trip brought fun back into my life. I had a blast hanging out with Derek and Gena. We attended a cold Baltimore Orioles game, watched *Dancing with the Stars* (a show I had never seen and may never watch again), went to eat at really cool restaurants, and just went for long, enjoyable walks around the Inner Harbor. Derek was nice enough to take off a couple of days to show me around the city. I told him I wanted to visit the aquarium that Denise and I always talked about seeing. Since Derek had already been there a number of times, he took care of some work business while I went to the aquarium by myself.

Derek had done a wonderful job of showing me how to get to the aquarium on one of those lengthy walks when we talked about our jobs and life in general. It was fairly easy walking over there that morning. I had my iPod on and enjoyed the time strolling over before the aquarium opened.

I always had a great time going to zoos and aquariums with Denise. I wasn't sure how I would respond visiting the aquarium without her. Getting there early turned out to be a smart move. I was one of the first people in line and to get into the first exhibit. I started to get really emotional and ended up having to walk away as fast as I could so that I didn't cry in front of other people. I felt deeply saddened by the thought of not being able to share this experience with Denise. The sense of loneliness and sorrow was overwhelming, and I didn't want to make a scene.

I knew Denise would have been impressed with the aquarium; our children would have loved it. The feeling of what could have been left me with such a sense of loss.

I got some lunch and handled myself better than I usually did, probably because I had already had my emotional moment. After I viewed all the exhibits, I headed out and returned to Derek's house. When I got back, I decided I would write some postcards until Derek and Gena arrived home.

The trip brought some happiness back into my life, and I felt lucky to have had the chance to visit and spend time with these dear friends. They were and are a loving family; soon their house would be a little livelier with the addition of their new little girl.

On the last morning, Derek and I went to eat breakfast before I dropped him off at the airport. Derek was going on a work trip and needed to get a rental car from the airport, so that is where we parted company; it didn't go so well.

I had an amazing time with him and Gena, laughing, cracking jokes, and just feeling happy. It was all coming to an end as I tearfully hugged Derek. This occasion was probably the most I have ever cried at an airport. Derek quickly could tell how difficult it was for me; he was really wonderful, telling me how nice it was to have me visit and how we would talk by phone. He also said he would continue to want to know how I was doing. But like all good things, this visit had come to an end.

I finally thanked Derek one last time for the escape from reality, but we both knew what came next. I had to drive home to a house that was empty and a reminder that six months ago I lost pretty much my whole world.

After Derek walked away, I sat in my car and uncontrollably cried. Even I didn't expect to be as emotional as I was. I will never forget that moment or the sad reality of the life I was about to walk back into.

The car ride home had much less traffic than the journey there. I was able to make it back to continue living in this disappointing world that I called my life. It took a couple of days to get back to my normal routines, but I managed. I had made it through six months. As much as that might seem to be a good thing, I remained in a state of profound grief, barely hanging on from day to day. Denise was in heaven with the babies, and I was still here on Earth, trying to hold on long enough until things got better. Then once things got better, I would have to live a second life, which I didn't want to live, because Denise and those kids were no longer with me. I felt pathetic.

Chapter 11

Six-Month Support

Ever since the first day of this tragedy, I had put a number of support pieces in place. I don't exactly know why I was able to think so rationally early on, but I suspect it was a benefit of being shocked and completely unprepared. As a result, it wasn't until a week after Denise and the babies' passing that things really started to sink in. Once I made it to the 6-month mark, I had to try to figure out which things I would keep in place and what activities I would need to start pulling away from.

The first and probably the best thing I did was to begin journaling and writing to Denise every night. I did this from the very first night of the tragedy for the next six months. I had no idea early on how long I would write to her, but I wanted to journal daily to keep her memory alive. I wrote at least a full page each night on a yellow legal pad, which was a little lengthy to continue doing that often. I didn't mind ending my night with my writing, but I recognized that it took quite some time. For a while, I thought it would have been quicker to type my thoughts and my daily activities but decided against it. After six months, I had to consider whether or not this was something I could maintain.

I knew I wouldn't be able to continue many of the coping strategies I had put in place and realized I would have to step away from some of these activities and at some point get on with the next phase of my life. The daily journaling seemed to be the first thing I could let go. Since I was with Derek and Gena at the six-month point, I decided I wouldn't finish my writings until the end of April, which would have been about a week later.

I struggled through the last week of my writing, knowing it would soon come to an end. I had become accustomed to ending every day composing to the woman I loved and always will love. However, I understood that writing to her every night was not something I could do for the rest of my life. I would pen my final letter on the last day of April. I grew more unsettled as the week progressed. I hated the fact that I was about to release this means of connection with the beautiful wife I loved. As I wrote my final "nightly reflections," those letters to Denise, I did so with a lump in my throat and tears in my eyes.

I loved Denise so dearly and this was my first step in trying to live without her in my life. I hated the feeling of letting go of this, but I knew that it was something I needed to do. I was lucky enough to realize early on the importance of carrying on her legacy and writing as therapy but understood that I had to relinquish it. As April came to a close, so did my daily journaling. The last letter I composed to her always will be one of the hardest things I ever wrote.

My next step was to determine another activity to help keep the memory of Denise alive. An idea came to me: I would use the same legal paper to list all the things I wanted to remember, in order, and write something about each one. I would tell our love story. I soon realized how lucky we were to have our photo albums and pictures saved on our phones and computer. We saved tickets from all the movies and sporting events and places we went together. I had spent time putting everything in order.

On that first day of May, I started telling our story from falling in love up until our very last night together. Even though I knew I would continue ending my days with thoughts of Denise, I still missed writing to her. But this was a logical step toward moving on with my life.

I had read a lot of books about overcoming grief and about heaven. Soon after her passing, I sought as many of these volumes as I could find, trying to consume different views, stories, and thoughts about how to manage this overwhelming sadness. When I got to the six-month mark, I thought this could be another activity to let go, but I knew I wasn't ready yet. I still struggled with managing my emotions and realized I would need to continue my nightly reading to better help me handle my feelings.

The next activity that I had built into my structure was a really difficult one. Every Sunday after church— even on those occasions when I was visiting a friend—I watched the film that Dawn and Brian had made for Denise's viewing. It was a half hour video of pictures set to Jason Mraz' music, and it was beautiful, wonderful, and horrible. I had watched it every Sunday.

Brian had kindly uploaded it to the internet and gave me the website so that even when I was out of town I could view it on my computer. It was painful to watch and made many of those Sundays much sadder, but it was a great way to program my brain to remember the good times. When I considered giving up this practice, I knew I wasn't ready. Watching the video would need to continue as it helped me remember the happy moments Denise and I shared.

The last piece of the structure I grappled with was by far the most difficult: my wedding ring. A number of the books I'd read by people who dealt with the same issue discussed how long to wear the wedding ring. I tried to take it off at the six-month mark, but, like some of my other support mechanisms, I knew I couldn't let go of this one. It was clear that I would take it off at some point, but I still needed to wear it. I still used "us" to describe Denise and me in conversations. My expressions had yet to catch up to the reality of my life. I recognized that I would need to take the ring off at some point. However, it wasn't going to be then.

Near the beginning of May, Bill, Judy, and I attended another evening dinner that was both beautiful and tragic. Since Denise was awarded the Teacher of the Year at her school, she was invited to the Teacher of the Year banquet that Raleigh hosts. Since Denise would not be able to attend, we were given the choice to go in her place. Bill, Judy, and I agreed to go, and I was very curious to see how I would handle this unique situation. I had no idea if anything was going to be said or if Denise was even going to come up. Either way I was fully prepared for a difficult evening.

I had talked to Bill and Judy about getting there early because I realized it would take time for me to get myself together. Also, I didn't want my emotional state to take any of the attention away from the people who were being honored. As we arrived, I was asked my name. The nice lady who checked us in understood the situation as soon as I answered. She checked us in and let me know she was one of the people who knew why Denise would not be attending. We went upstairs and there were a lot of smiles and people taking pictures. I just tried to get out of the way and waited until the doors were opened to get my head where it needed to be to handle the evening as best as I could.

Before the doors opened, one of Denise's cousins came to check on me. Rick was a principal at another Raleigh school and probably one of the coolest people I have ever met. He sat with me and asked how I was doing.

"If you need anything, I'm here," Rick said. "I know this can't be easy. I'll help you through it in any way I can."

Once the doors opened, Rick and I walked in followed closely by Bill and Judy. Rick and I soon realized that our tables were right next to each other, which was going to help a great deal. I found our table and sat down.

I had previously attended a Teacher of the Year banquet when I first met Denise, and I was presented with a little clear award to congratulate me on representing our school as the Teacher of the Year. I knew there was likely to be a similar award for Denise. But I was not prepared for the words "In Memory of" before her name.

I was so much on edge by the time we actually took our seats that I felt I needed to get out of the big banquet hall as quickly as I could. Since we were among the first people in the room, I was able to leave without causing a scene. I found a place in the corner and just sat and cried.

It took me a fair amount of time before I was ready to return and sit with Bill and Judy. Once I was better able to handle the situation, I went back to my seat. Bill and Judy asked how I was.

"I just wasn't expecting the words 'In Memory of' to be put on her award," I said. "It was probably the right thing for them to do, but I just never would have imagined us talking about Denise in the past tense."

It still seemed so wrong. I started looking at the other information on the table and spotted a brochure that listed all the Teacher of the Year representatives. As I scrolled through the list, I saw all the names of people, and, sure enough, once again the words "In Memory of" appeared in front of Denise's name. I had to exit the banquet hall again, find my corner and cry some more.

Tears flowed down my cheeks many times that evening, but crying was normal under the circumstances. This tragedy never should have happened. I was so unprepared for it and all that followed. After that second set of tears, I was able to cope better. There was one other time I needed to leave when I ended up talking with Rick outside the banquet hall.

I will never forget that evening for a variety of reasons. It was another of those experiences I had to face without the woman I loved.

With the Teacher of the Year banquet behind me, it was time to get back to things that were easier to deal with. Unfortunately, the "year of firsts" was about to strike again, but this time we were all better prepared.

Denise's family and I had talked about how we were going to deal with Mother's Day. We agreed we would go to the beach for the weekend to get away from the reality we were facing. Denise's family, including Brian's parents, got a beach house for the weekend, and we all had a lovely time. Dawn and Brian found a place with most of the bedrooms downstairs and the master bedroom, kitchen, and living room upstairs. Being with family helped us get through an otherwise challenging holiday. We walked a lot, ate out at various restaurants, and even spent a morning at the beach playing around. We found a loving way to deal with the sadness that Mother's Day brought us that year.

As the "year of firsts" continued, I approached our first wedding anniversary that I would spend alone. I visited Denise's niche as I had on most of the other important days. I bought a card and read it to her. My sad reality slowly became the norm. I was far from numb as I sat at her niche on those special days, but I had done it enough to better understand how to handle those occasions. You never get used to spending such moments in front of your wife and children's urn instead of seeing them in person.

In early June, Denise's family and I went to her school for a dedication. Her principal, PTA, parents, and everyone at the school were so gracious to all of us during those tough times. They treated us with such care. However, this trip resulted in large part from the efforts of another organization.

While Denise was pregnant and trying to work on her maternity lesson plans, on several Sunday mornings we visited her school to get some materials from her classroom. We learned that a local church used their facilities during those early Sunday mornings. Apparently one of the members who attended those services heard about Denise's passing and wanted to do something to honor her. The gesture was all the more amazing since I don't believe the church members ever even met Denise.

The church purchased a bench and donated it to the school in remembrance of Denise. They positioned it in the back where most of the teachers watched their students during recess. It was a considerate tribute, and the dedication ceremony was meaningful. I talked to a couple of the people whom I recognized, and Denise's amazing principal said a few words. Then everyone planted seeds around the outside by the fence. It was a loving way for the school and church to commemorate one its shining stars.

The bench was a beautiful piece of craftsmanship and featured a plaque with Denise's name and the babies' names, something I didn't expect but greatly appreciated. It was a picturesque spot for a beautiful bench in a world that continued to be dark.

As the unrelenting "year of firsts" progressed, we got closer and closer to Denise's birthday. I had been preparing for this day for over two months. I have to give credit to Dawn for first putting the idea in my head.

Right after Denise passed, when the investigator had first told Bill, Judy, Dawn, and me that she died quickly, Dawn mentioned that I should think about holding a 5K race in her honor. She said that even though Denise wasn't a big runner, she was proud that I enjoyed jogging so much. I was acquainted with many people who had put on 5K races and knew a fair amount about these events.

Since we already had a memorial fund and people were generous in their giving, we figured this might be an annual event that we could use to support the cause. Dawn and I already had given checks from our memorial fund to the four schools where Denise taught so they could order new books for their libraries. We also donated to the Girls on the Run program, which Denise was a part of, and a couple other organizations that Denise believed in.

For the longest time, I didn't have much that kept me looking forward. I spent the first couple of months completely in survival mode. The thought that we might be able to hold this race became a reality. Early on I told Dawn the first thing we needed was a place to run and a race logo. If we could get those two things, we had a starting point. Dawn had tried to find someone to create a logo but we initially had no success.

During one of my visits to my neighbors, I told Adam's wife Tricia what we were trying to do, and she asked if she could give it a shot. I was more than happy to have her come up with a logo that would be imprinted on all of the race materials. If we could get a logo, we would be one huge step closer to making the race happen.

I gave Tricia some of Denise's pictures and my notes about what I was looking for. She and Adam stopped over one afternoon and showed me what she and another person had put together, a beautiful caricature-style picture, and it brought me to tears. I was so honored that Tricia did such a great job with it. She took my notes and made it a reality.

I really wanted the logo to include Denise's beautiful smile and the fact that she was a big proponent of wearing scarves as well as being a teacher. The logo consisted of a beautiful smile, a scarf, and one shoulder holding a bag with a ruler sticking out of it with a book in the other hand. I told Tricia and Adam how much I loved the logo and how it was the first big hurdle we needed to climb for our 5K race.

The next step was trying to find a place to run. Since we were going to attempt to hold the race around her birthday, June 21, there wasn't going to be too much time to run on a street. There are a number of road races, and I wanted to do something different, so I came up with the idea of racing at a park that I drove by daily on the way to work. The natural setting was ideal for walking or running. I didn't know if they would let me conduct the race there, but the least I could do was ask.

Sadly, I was told that I probably wasn't going to be able to hold the event there. I received a couple of other suggestions, but I wanted to make the race special and was afraid I wasn't going to be able to accomplish that goal.

Every once in a while, people come into your life whom you will never forget. I was about to meet a couple of these wonderful people. At school, because of the large number of special education students we had, we were able to hire a part-time special education teacher. As a school, we decided it would be best to have someone every day for the last five months of the school year rather than bringing in a teacher only a couple of days a week for much longer. This approach gave us more time to find the ideal person for the job.

Enter Ando Huffman. Mrs. Huffman was a substitute and taught at our school a couple of times. After a few conversations with her, I thought she was wonderful. She cared deeply about the kids and seemed to do amazingly well when she subbed in the special education classroom. One afternoon as the students were getting ready for dismissal, I talked with her and learned that she had her degree in special education.

I instantly thought, "Man, I wish we could hire her; she is great!"

The next day when I mentioned to Mrs. Ring, one of the other special education teachers, that Mrs. Huffman had her degree in special education, Mrs. Ring informed me that we might have some employment months of pay to hire additional help. Sure enough, after interviewing for the position, Mrs. Huffman got the job.

Mrs. Huffman filtered in and out of some of the higher needs classes, which had the most special education students. Since I had some of the bigger classes of fourth and fifth graders, I was able to get to work with Mrs. Huffman daily. We became good friends. She knew of my story and, as a person that exercises regularly and enjoys running, she seemed to take an interest in my idea of putting on a race.

Luckily for me, Ando had connections. One day Mrs. Huffman mentioned that I should sit down with her husband Adam and have a conversation. I was all for such a discussion and I was able to speak to Mrs. Huffman's wonderful husband, a parks and recreation employee. Mr. Huffman cared about my current situation and seemed to want to try to help any way he could. I think he understood how much this possible race meant to me. I was hoping he could recommend potential places for the event. He did one better. He informed me there was a chance I could hold it in the park I wanted to use. Because this was going to be the first time they tried to run a 5K around that park, he said I would need to do a lot of planning in order to make it work.

I was thrilled by this possibility. Making all the necessary preparations became therapy for me. I was more than willing to put in the effort. I considered all the different aspects of the race. The park service went above and beyond in order to help me reach my goal. I will forever be grateful for everyone involved who gave me a chance to do something good and an avenue to keep moving forward as well as a way I could heal by carrying on Denise's legacy.

I still had a lot of sad and angry thoughts that I wanted to replace by focusing my attention on making this the best event possible. I felt excited by every inch of progress towards my goal. With both the logo and the race location achieved, what remained was getting everything else together.

One of the sad realities of my life was that I spent so much time alone. Putting on a race was probably difficult with a family, especially if you are doing it for the first time. There are a lot of smart people who hold these kinds of events, but I was coming from a much different angle. On Sundays after walking with Mr. Bob, I spent hours sitting on the couch putting together paperwork, writing proposals, sending emails, and making notes about everything that needed to be done. It was a welcome escape from my normal thoughts, a way to fill my time and occupy my mind with something much more constructive.

The family certainly stepped up to help. Dawn got the brochures created and the T-shirts organized. Bill and Judy spoke to a number of restaurants and companies in the area about sponsoring. We were all given the chance to work together to honor Denise's memory. It was gratifying to work together to create a way to remember the very best of Denise.

I hated that Denise was gone, but under the circumstances I knew this was the best way to deal with the overwhelming loss we suffered. A lot of people helped organize the event in her memory. I will forever recall those kind souls who gave me a chance to carry on Denise's legacy while doing something good and continuing my healing process. We had been given a tragic set of circumstances. We all tried to find the best way to live and work in this new reality that we faced.

Chapter 12

The 5K Run for Dee Dee

Years from now when I look back on my life, I think my two greatest accomplishments will be (1) surviving after the loss of my wife and babies and (2) putting on that race. I will be proud of that 5K race for the rest of my life. But the sad truth of it is I wish I never had needed to put it on.

Before the race happened, I needed to celebrate Denise's birthday the only way I knew how. As I did for all holidays and special events, I sat at her niche, talking to her. I read the birthday card I got for her, crying as I uttered each word.

Every morning I awakened to this reality without Denise. Every evening I went home to that empty house. It was what it was.

That year she would have been 40 years old. Like all the holidays that had passed over the months since her passing, she should have been there to celebrate her birthday with two screaming babies at her side. That would have been the best present Denise ever received. But that was not the case. Denise and those babies were up in heaven while the rest of us here on Earth thought of them constantly.

Thankfully, the race was close to occupy some of my time and my thoughts. Otherwise, I may not have made it through her birthday as well as I did. Very early on, we as a family spoke about doing the race in late June because her birthday was the 21st. We figured it would help us through the grief, and, even though late June might be sweltering, holding the race then would give us a sense of purpose. The family definitely were right about that.

A number of people helped with the race preparations. My Dad, who knew how much this event meant to me both as a person trying to do something good and as someone who was still grieving, came over about ten days before the race. I showed him all the materials we had, and he did an amazing job of helping to organize things while I was at work. Looking back on it, I don't know if I would have been ready without his help. I probably should have taken some time off to get everything together. Since I continued to teach, Dad's help proved invaluable in getting ready for the race. Every day when I came home, he showed me what he had accomplished. He did a wonderful job of sorting through all the participant race shirts and volunteer race shirts, getting the packet pickup bags together, and even helping a great deal with the timing equipment.

Bill and Judy were in charge of the food table and were thoroughly prepared. They provided a large amount of the bottled water, which each participant would receive after they crossed the finish line. They came over one afternoon and worked with dad to put all the participant packets together. Judy had the brilliant idea of using gallon-size Ziploc bags so that everything was prepared and easy to see.

The company that helped our participants have exact race times was easy to work with. The company consisted of some of my old friends with whom I used to run the streets of Rocky Mount, North Carolina, years before I met Denise. In fact, one of the timing people, Michael, went to Oregon to run the marathon with Derek and me one year. The other, Scott, was in a 200-mile relay event with me while I attended grad school. Both Michael and Scott were great to work with. Although they had never met Denise, they could see how much she had meant to me. Michael and Scott's help made the race a much better experience. Having two old friends there with me made a huge difference.

We had an amazing number of volunteers, people who weren't runners but believed in what we were trying to do. I met some wonderful helpers the week before the race who let me show them where I was going to put them on the course. A couple of them had no idea what they were getting into when they signed up, and I pretty much forgot how long the walk was to some of their course spots. A large number of volunteers checked people in. Even a couple of my students showed up to help pass out water to all the finishing participates.

Denise's principal wanted to play a part in the race and agreed to organize the water station. All the volunteers had their own special T-shirts, but at the water station many of the volunteers from the school where Denise taught sported their school T-shirts to honor her.

We were all fortunate that we received the okay to run around the property and that the staff at the park was obliging in organizing the Porta Potties, tables, and parking, and even making sure that the grass was cut. The race course was just as I had hoped it would be.

Mr. Bob and I walked the path weekly in anticipation of the upcoming event. I was worried about snakes, so, to put my mind at ease, I decided to run the course at the 7:00 a.m. start time for two Saturdays prior to the event. Luckily, I didn't see any snakes. A great medic who had heard about the race remained on hand for the event just in case. He appreciated being a part of the event, and his presence there meant the world to me.

We started the race pretty early to accommodate the park since they were being more than cooperative with us.

Someone who wasn't even in attendance aided our efforts tremendously. Because we have this memorial fund through the community foundation, much of the paperwork I needed to complete was filtered through a wonderful person named Quinn. Words can't describe how wonderful she was at helping with all the insurance, the website, and ordering the T-shirts and awards. Her overall support meant a great deal. Without her help and that of the employees who were responsible for our fund, the race would not have been as successful as it was.

The race got off to a less than stellar start. The evening before the race we had set up some time for packet pickup and registration. I was a bit tardy to packet pickup because

I learned late that, although I thought we were ready with our water stations, some uncertainty still existed. After I met with Denise's principal and talked her through everything, we were all set. However, that put me behind in arriving for packet pickup. I had all of the participant's packets, and, since I was running a little late, a number of questions arose about how to set up the tables and chairs.

When I got to the park, I apologized for my tardiness and explained how to set everything up. The family brought up a couple questions and suggestions, which were good points. However, I wanted everything to be organized as it would be the next day and had already turned in a sight map with the setup. I was concerned that if this didn't go well and I wasn't prepared for some part of the race, the park might not let us hold the race there in the future. Some questions and concerns remained, but I cordially encouraged everyone to follow my lead regarding the arrangements. Some tensions surfaced, and I didn't handle myself as well as I would have hoped. Thankfully, people were already showing up to volunteer and pick up their packets, so things calmed down.

One thing I didn't consider fully was the heat and sun. I didn't have any tents, but luckily Brian was able to provide one. Dad grabbed me some food before I arrived, and I ate as I got everything in place and showed people where I would have them the next day.

I spent much of my time walking people to where they would be the following morning and little on check in. The volunteers working with the packet pickup handled that beautifully. After preparations at the venue were completed, Dad and I headed home to do some additional work. It took us a while to get everything finalized for the next morning, which would come quickly.

I slept poorly that night and not simply from nerves preceding the race. Some anger about how things were handled when I showed up late lingered.

I had studied the weather forecast religiously and thought we were going to be dry. *Thought* being the key word. Morning came early and Dad and I put everything together and headed out in the darkness. As we drove to the park, heavy rain began to pour. Tears washed down my cheeks as I drove. I couldn't believe the rain might ruin an event we had worked so hard to bring to fruition. Luckily it stopped by the time we got to the park and my tears dried up as well.

The morning went well. Seeing all the people who showed up to support what I felt was a great cause warmed my heart. Thanks to the rain, a rainbow appeared, which made everyone including me smile. A couple of the volunteers took a picture of the race sign with the rainbow. That will probably always be one of my favorite pictures.

Although the rain had made me sad and nervous, it turned out to be a gift. In addition to the rainbow, the rain alleviated some of the heat and humidity, so the weather was wonderful. After I worked so diligently and poured my heart into making the event successful, I felt gratified and relieved.

Some attendees drove over three hours to volunteer. Dad was out in the parking lot helping people park their vehicles. A number of my colleagues from school donated their time to check people in. Even some of my former students agreed to come be a part of the event that I had worked so hard to put together.

During the introductions, I had no idea what to say about why we all had gathered for the race. I said something along the lines of us joining together for a reason that was difficult, and I left it at that.

A great group of participants of all ages and sizes took part in the race. My goal for the event was to provide a fun environment for people of all ages. A large number of children and many retirees participated. I dreamed that this race would welcome people who didn't normally get out and exercise; based on the number of kids and the large contingency of Bill and Judy's retired friends, I feel that we achieved something special.

I had everything planned ahead of time. That morning from the moment I stepped out of my car, I was moving. It was an emotional day but, because I was so active, I handled it as well as I could have. The first time I took a really deep breath was during the National Anthem. Luckily everyone was turned toward the flag, and only those standing next to me saw me begin to tear up. I was able to get myself together enough toward the end of the song to start the race. After that, I went back to moving and taking care of all the responsibilities I had as organizer.

As the race started, I looked out across the crowd of people who had come to be a part of Denise's legacy. The race course was not easy. Mr. Bob and I spent a great deal of time trying to find the best place to run. I hoped to get people spaced out enough so that they wouldn't be bunched together on the trail, and going around the beautiful lake. Luckily, the field the participants ran around first seemed to separate people enough so there were no issues. Seeing all the runners dashing along the trail gave me hope that I could function as an adult, even in my current state. With a lot of help from family and friends, I had somehow managed to bring this dream to life. More than anything, that gave me hope for the future.

The race went over well and everyone seemed to have fun. One of my student's families showed up out of the blue and asked if they could help. We got their kids to pass out water. It was such a beautiful event and a wonderful day that I was so fortunate to be a part of.

It was a joy to witness so many people of different ages participating. Bill and Judy invited a large number of people from their retiree group, so there was quite a contingent of participants over 50 and active. Not all of them ran; some walked. Seeing a couple of people cross the finish line with their walkers brought a warmness to my heart. One lady who couldn't make it all the way around the lake, so she got a golf cart ride to the finish line where she crossed and was cheered on.

The crowd was comprised of people I knew, some I had seen before, and many whom I had never met, and I wouldn't have wanted it any other way. The police investigator whom I'll always remember had never run a race, but he participated and appeared to have a good time. Gordon, the man who married Denise and me, drove all the way from his home in Virginia with one of his daughters just to support us. The best and most memorable individual was my wonderful former student Davis, who had passed out bulletins at our wedding. He had a blast while being pushed in his wheelchair by a couple of men, who seemed to go much faster with Davis than I would have been able to run myself.

Overall it was a spectacular event. We held awards and rewarded the fastest of the fast. I tried to say everyone's name correctly and think I did a good enough job. Mrs. Huffman and her two amazing kids helped me pass out the awards. It turned out to be a wonderful day that I will never forget.

The event went off without any big issues. Everyone seemed to have a good time aiding a worthy cause, and everybody was safe.

Afterward, many of the runners and volunteers stayed to help clean up. At the end everyone went back to their lives hopefully with smiles on their faces.

Before the event, I had the idea that I would run the course myself after everyone left. It would be my way of participating and also a chance to make sure there wasn't any trash left behind. As good as the park was to us, I wanted to be certain we kept it as clean as it was before we started our race. I also hoped we would be given the opportunity to hold the race there again the following year.

A couple of my best friends, William and Anthony Lucas, came over for the race. While we were cleaning up, I mentioned to them that if they would want to stay till the end, I was going to run the course and they were more than welcome to join me. Sure enough, those fast friends waited until everyone left and ran with me at a much slower pace than they had earlier in the day. The Lucases were great and I always will believe it would have been perfect to have our boy named Lucas, even if he never developed the way he should.

I won't lie, the course was hard; I knew that, and I didn't pace myself enough and had to do a little bit of walking coming up the tough final hill. I didn't really mind as I was just happy that everything turned out as well as it did.

The best part of the race was that so many people participated in the day and even in the preparations beforehand. Every person who attended or even just donated was responsible for how successful that race turned out to be.

I felt conflicted because, on the one hand, I was delighted the race went so well, but, on the other hand, I desperately wished we never needed to hold it.

I was pleased with the final outcome. Looking back on it, I don't think it could have been any more perfect than it was.

Back home Dad and I talked at length about how well we thought everything turned out. We were both so gratified by the success but agreed that future events might never be as good as that first year. Honestly, I'm okay with that. The race was a big part of my healing and grieving. It gave me hope to keep going and a goal to work toward, and it all worked out in the end. The race may never again be as good as that day's event, but I feel that everyone who was there and joined in the experience will always remember it and be proud they were a part of it.

Dad and I relaxed some more and cleaned up a lot of the stuff that we used. For dinner we went to Dawn and Brian's, had pizza and hung out with family. We talked a good deal about how successful we felt the race was. Hearing other people express how well they thought everything was prepared and how they enjoyed the morning brought a sense of comfort and satisfaction. People had offered me so much support, and I really hoped I was able to give them back something while still trying to mourn and grieve as I was. The race was wonderful for so many reasons, and the worst part of the day was the realization that it was all over.

Dad and I had discussions about what was going to happen when the race ended and how I would be able to cope with the fact that I didn't have this to think about any more. It wasn't something I was looking forward to, but my biggest fear was how I would handle it if this race wasn't successful. Fortunately, there were no injuries and everyone seemed to have a really good time, which put my biggest fear at ease. However, I remained concerned about the letdown afterward being tough for me. During the week of preparation before the event, my life was filled with activity to focus my thoughts, and Dad was with me. He would be leaving the following Monday, and the empty life I didn't want was still going to be there waiting for me. I still faced a number of challenges ahead and hoped I wouldn't get more negativity to add to the depression I might enter after the race was behind me.

As successful as the 5K was, and it was a day I will never forget, we all knew I was about to go over a metaphorical cliff. The fall would speak to how well my healing was progressing. I hoped that the letdown after the conclusion of the race was the only challenge ahead. Unfortunately, I had more troubles looming.

Chapter 13

Medical

There was a massive aspect to Denise's passing that I had been trying to deal with since the unfortunate events that now overshadowed my life. The fact was that a 39-year-old, "at-risk" patient who had been seen by two different doctors the week before her passing had died. Based on the medical examiner's report, Denise passed away due of "an acute intracerebral (brain) hemorrhage originating in an area consistent with hypertensive etiology" (high blood pressure). Our two beautiful, healthy children left this world with her.

Those were the facts. However, I held certain beliefs that contributed considerably to my current state of mind. One of the issues plaguing me stemmed from seeing how unhappy my wife was with the treatment from her OB/GYN. Unfortunately, because of my work schedule, I was never able to witness her treatment. My work had been kind enough to let me leave early on Wednesdays so I could meet Denise for her weekly prenatal appointment, which fell directly after her OB/GYN. I hadn't met the obstetric doctors who saw Denise and never witnessed how they treated her. But what I saw in Denise's face after those appointments will forever stick with me.

I knew in my heart that she probably wasn't being cared for with the Golden Rule in mind. Based on how she looked in the parking lot of the prenatal office on a number of occasions, it was clear that she probably wasn't given the respect an "at-risk" patient deserved, let alone a beautiful pregnant woman. Denise told me that she called and complained about her treatment after how those doctors made her feel. I believe she spoke to the office manager. Unfortunately, when sifting through her paperwork from the OB/GYN, I could find no documentation of such a phone call.

I had noticed a pattern but, reflecting back on it, I didn't give it the proper thought I should have. I knew how amazing our story was. I always believed in Karma and in God and believed in my heart that our fairytale would end with us holding those precious babies and living happily ever after. We had been through so much that our ending had to be a happy one. I felt that, if she wasn't being treated to the best of those doctor's abilities, it was just another obstacle Denise and I would face on our quest to be the family we always dreamed we would be.

I had put my trust in God and the medical community as a whole to give us what we had worked so hard for, and I just assumed the doctors, even those without the greatest bedside manner, would soon become a part of our past that we would joke about as our kids grew up. Never in a million years would I understand that a simple mistake would be the difference between a doctor with bad bedside manner and poor medical care.

When Denise and the babies first passed, I was in shock as I spoke with the investigator whose job it was to make sure I had nothing to do with her death. I didn't believe I could live without Denise. I explained to the investigator how hard it would be to go on without her. Beyond that, what I couldn't live with more than Denise, was the thought that this could happen to someone else if I didn't do everything I could to make sure it didn't. That guilt would eat away at me daily for the rest of my life. No one should feel the type of pain I experienced then. That belief drove me to fight the injustice that I believe this tragedy was.

During the period of shock after Denise first passed, I was still worried about other people. I was proud of myself for wanted to protect others from this kind of heartbreak.

As I look back, I realize I hadn't hit the anger stage yet. I was about to lose much of my rationality. The shock of her death had made my mind more focused on trying to do my part to help others rather than worrying about the next stage of grief.

I have never been an angry person. Some things can get under my skin. Disrespect aggravates me. I try to teach my students to treat everyone with respect. They still sometimes try my patience in this regard, but they are kids and always learning. My students are there to get an education, and I am responsible for teaching them. I can forgive a lack of regard in children, but I expect respect from adults. Before this happened, I would have said rudeness irritated me more than most anything else. That was before my entire world crumbled.

When my shock transformed into anger, I was unprepared for the level of rage I never knew I was capable of. I hated what had happened and wanted someone to answer for what clearly was a mistake. Her OB/GYN was paid to look after her health. She was "at-risk" and more than 36 weeks pregnant when she died. I didn't understand why she was allowed to continue to carry the babies to labor when she was worried about her health. If there was a .0001% chance of this happening, a C-section to deliver those babies should have been conducted.

Of course, like the Monday morning quarterback, hindsight allows for a clearer view. I look back at all of this through the lens of how things ended. That may not be fair, but it was my reality.

It was challenging to process a level of anger I had never experienced. Frankly, I was furious and I had every right to be. If this had occurred four or five months into the pregnancy, this tragedy could not have been avoided. However, at nine months pregnant, this could and most assuredly *should* have been prevented.

These thoughts and feelings plagued my sleep many nights. While the sleep meds thankfully knocked me out, they could not keep me asleep. If I had to get up to go to the bathroom in the middle of the night, I knew I wasn't going back to sleep. Rage acts like a stimulant, not a sedative. It took some time but I eventually adjusted my dinner schedule to account for this fact. I tried to finish eating by 6:30 p.m. in hopes that I wouldn't need to awaken to use the bathroom.

It was really difficult to stop thinking about the obvious medical mistake long enough to fall asleep. I couldn't understand how this happened. Because of the constant anger, I clenched my teeth without even realizing it, so much so that my jaw would hurt even at school. I kept a scowl on my face because of the anger that was deep inside. I learned that I needed to drink a lot of water to alleviate the headaches I was getting. All this because I was enraged, and I had plenty to fuel my anger.

One night while I was brushing my teeth, Denise had told me she didn't think she could go the last two weeks of her pregnancy. I reminded her of all those people who weren't able to get to that point. I believed that everything would turn out the way it was supposed to. I was so blinded by my belief in our happy ending that I was completely unprepared for her passing.

At a certain point, as most people would, I started questioning my role in Denise's death. I played everything over again and again in my mind through the lens of the ending. I came to realize I was an enabler. I had allowed those doctors to treat her the way they did because I had kept my mouth shut and didn't speak up for her. I have always felt that one of my greatest strengths was being able to handle situations the correct way. However, by not speaking up, I was permitting the doctors to continue her treatment as it was. I assumed everything would turn out the way it was meant to. I failed my wife when she needed me most, and that will haunt me until I join her in heaven.

Around Christmas Denise's family and I sought legal representation. Dawn had heard about a gentlemen who agreed to help us get the answers we so desperately needed. Unfortunately, he was unable to take the case, and he informed us of some sad truths. He said the earlier we learned them, the better our understanding of the whole situation would be.

He explained that, although Denise carried two healthy full-term babies inside her, this would be viewed as one death. That shook me to my core. I couldn't believe that in these types of circumstances the babies didn't matter in a court of law. Many times I had heard all the arguments on abortion and understood both sides of the issue. However, this policy seemed horrible and wrong and completely disrespectful to people living through the aftermath of such a tragedy. Sometimes things don't make sense, and this rule is one of them. But I had to come to grips with the fact that I would need to take my emotions out of this to better understand all the things we as a family were up against.

This lawyer was a good man, but it took a long time to hear from him. I spent too many sleepless, empty nights waiting to get closure. When the decision finally came, he was not able to find someone that could take Denise's case. This dead end hit me hard. That night I called Mr. Bob and Dad to talk to both of them. It seemed so wrong on so many levels.

In the long run, the attorney's honesty was what we needed, even though it was hard to hear. I have believed for the longest time that I was willing to take the harder road as long as it ended up where I needed to be. This was another example of that belief. The process of trying to bring closure to our unique situation took much longer than anyone would have wished, but as a result I was much better able to handle the reality the lawyer shared. So much time had passed between the initial meeting and him informing us that he wasn't able to provide legal counsel, I was better prepared to handle that disappointing news.

I still had a huge amount of anger and was aware that I wasn't managing everything as well as I wanted. I had to wrap my brain around what all of this meant and see the big picture. I hated the fact that the legal side of all of this meant that I was viewed as a possible lawsuit plaintiff rather than a person grieving, but clearly law wasn't written for me. The sooner I realized that, the fewer sleepless nights I would have.

As mentioned earlier, the way I viewed what happened was that, if this occurred when Denise was four or five months pregnant, it was God's doing. If this took place six months into the pregnancy, it was still likely God acting, but a medical mistake may have contributed. At seven months, although the Divine may have played a part, medical mistakes were more likely. If Denise had passed at eight months, it was probably the result of a medical error and less probable that God played a hand. But nine months into a pregnancy it seems almost certain that malpractice was to blame.

Those babies were ready to arrive, and the amount of stress on Denise's body could have removed and would have been warranted. If we had ended up in the hospital and this still had happened, I could have slept better knowing that we at least made it there. I'm sure I will always wonder what would have happened if the babies were delivered earlier, but under the circumstances I had enough anger to process.

If I had felt she was given the best treatment, I think I would have managed the anger better.

Not long after the 5k event, these issues arose when I had a phone appointment with the next lawyer whom I asked to look at the information. He came highly recommended, and I was impressed when I first met with him. He was honest and compassionate, and I felt very comfortable with him.

As with the previous attorney, he informed me that there wasn't enough information to warrant him taking the case. I was dumbfounded. As I navigated the letdown after the race, this blow hit me hard. It seemed that in the grand scheme of life no one cared about Denise's passing. Her death was just going away as if it didn't matter. No one would care 20 years from now that it was wrong. The doctors would continue to mistreat their patients and probably get away with another tragedy like this.

During this period, some colleagues at work clearly recognized I was going through a tough time. Most people likely chalked it up to the race being over. While I definitely felt some depression after the event ended, that sadness was overshadowed by my anger and the fear that no one would learn from Denise's death and what was done to her easily could happen to someone else. It was a tough pill to swallow and, as painful as my life was up to that point, I reached a whole new level of sadness.

I thanked this lawyer for his honesty and tried to continue with my life such as it was, but clearly I wasn't who I once had been. Luckily most people attributed my deeper sorrow to the conclusion of the race. It was a wretched realization I was learning: The world didn't care about Denise, and Denise probably was better to this world than it was to her. I didn't know what to do.

Even with my emotional attachment, as time went on, I became better at understanding how this was viewed to outsiders. I had to grasp the very real possibility that there were questions I would never get answers to and that I might never get the type of closure I desperately needed.

The hardest aspect of trying to understand the medical issues of this came down to lacking enough data to prove those babies had to be removed. But I continued to struggle with why Denise's individual records were considered more important than the overall statistics about "at risk" pregnancies. She and I sat through multiple meetings about how she was an at-risk patient. We understood the dangers, but there was nothing Denise could have done differently. She shared her concerns twice the week before she passed only to have two different doctors send her out the door, telling her she would be fine.

I witnessed how she felt the last Wednesday at the prenatal visit. She was by far the most distressed I ever had seen her. It was extremely difficult to calm her down on the walk from the parking lot to the prenatal office. My biggest fear was always that her anxiety was going to affect the babies. In the end, looking back on it, we all should have listened to her.

I say we *all* should have listened because I'm not without some accountability. I was the enabler in this situation. I could have gone into the office and started cussing and flipping tables, and they still might have said she was fine. However, if I had been escorted out by some security guard or law enforcement, I would probably have slept more soundly after her passing, knowing that I didn't sit idly by when my wife needed me the most.

As the month progressed, I began to look more rationally at the situation and started realizing that it wasn't fair to blame the medical community as a whole. As the laws are written, these type of things are more prone to happen, but that's not fair to all the wonderful people in the medical community. It's possible the best of doctors would have made the same decision and had the same outcome. But I still have to live with the thought that maybe I should have done more. Had I really understood how much pain Denise was in?

There were some really good people in the medical community and I needed to do my part to reach out to them. I wrote to my own doctor and told her how much I appreciated her and apologized for not coming to see her. She cared deeply for me and was affected by Denise's passing. I sent a card to the prenatal office, whose staff went out of their way to support Denise and me both in her life and after her death. These were great people that cared and showed compassion.

I even wrote a letter to the one doctor at her OB/GYN who treated Denise as the queen she was. After she saw him, I could always tell because she was beaming when she left the office. I was even given the opportunity to speak to an OB/GYN who came to the house to hear my story, to see the pictures of Denise, and to try to help me better understand what happened.

Even in my darkest hour, I felt it was important to shine a light on the great people who actually helped us. I thanked each one of those kind souls who gave me hope in a time I felt so alone and lost. Even though the rules might not have been in my favor, there were people I could honestly thank. I took comfort in recognizing the caring, wonderful representatives of a community I had such anger toward.

I was disappointed at how I had handled things internally. I hoped very few people ever encountered the rawness I was going through.

After thanking the helpers I had encountered in the medical community, I wondered if I could do more by sharing my story to prevent others from experiencing similar tragedies. I sent an email to a couple of medical conferences to see if I could speak about Denise's passing and relay my message about listening to patients and treating them by following the Golden Rule. Sadly, I never heard back from them. Nonetheless, I was glad I reached out because at least it made me feel I was doing my part to encourage the kind of care that might have saved my wife and children. Three deaths were already too many not to learn something from this tragedy.

I made attempts to speak with less anger about what happened to us, but I still had to deal with intense emotions. Although it was an uncomfortable thought, I always wondered if the staff at that doctor's office might have preferred if I committed suicide. If I had died, those doctors would have had nothing to fear in the aftermath of Denise and those babies' deaths. The idea troubled me. I'm sure that most people go into the medical profession to help people, but they never reached out to me after Denise's passing when I so desperately needed them to. I'm sure they would not have wanted my suicide, but the nagging notion remained for some time.

Because I lived in the house by myself and have had a tendency to overanalyze, loved ones may well have been concerned that I would contemplate suicide. Without someone to keep me company, all I had were my thoughts, and the mind games I played brought many internal issues.

One of the realizations that I came to was this idea: I live with regret but not with guilt. I trusted the medical community and the doctors at her OB/GYN. I believed them and thought they knew best. I don't have a medical degree, so I put my faith in the people with those degrees and I lost. I live with regret that I didn't do more when I knew she was in pain and was worried about her safety. I sat in those at-risk meetings with her, and I am not totally innocent in Denise's death. I will always wish I had done more.

Trust comes with a lot of baggage. After everything that happened, I got a simple card from the OB/GYN and a refund for what ended up being the money that we proactively paid for the twins' delivery. Apart from that, I didn't hear from him. I understood why they never reached out to me because it was a legal issue. But the hardest part was the realizing the physicians I trusted with the person I loved most in this world cared more about themselves than they did for me after Denise died.

Many people told me that their lawyers had probably instructed them not to contact me. I'm quite sure those doctors felt remorse and suspected they wanted to do something to help me. But because they were told not to, they just let me be. My belief is that we could have found a middle ground.

Because I spent so much time alone, I became greatly bothered by this. If they had sent me a card and in it had simply written, "We think of you every day," that would have meant the world to me.

It was hard for me to fathom how a mistake like this happened and how the doctors and the office just moved on afterward. If I were in their shoes, I would have been devastated; I would have found it almost impossible to do my normal job.

I wouldn't want those doctors to stop working because then they couldn't help all the other pregnant women who rely on them like Denise and I did. However, if they had let me know they were thinking of me, I feel they could have done so without showing any guilt. My life was so empty, and I so desperately needed to know they cared about me. However, the rules are the rules, and clearly those rules weren't written for me.

I needed to have answers to my questions and I wasn't finding any. The closure I required in order to put Denise's death behind me may remain a door that will never be shut. I wouldn't wish this pain on anyone. The idea that it simply was what it was seems so wrong when I consider the type of person Denise was and the legacy she left. She deserved this world's best, but the world didn't live up to its end of the bargain. I will always wonder how our lives would have turned out differently.

I hoped this failure would not repeat itself after Denise's passing, but I understood there was a very real possibility it might continue. I know Denise would have been proud of me for deciding I didn't want to be part of the problem, that I was willing to be part of the solution. I think she would smile to know that I tried to hold them accountable for their actions out of a desire for patient prevention rather than revenge.

I encountered so many challenges that year. Denise and I almost had everything, but the cruel reality was we were totally unprepared for what the world had in store for us. I was equally unequipped as I searched for ways to turn Denise's death into a learning tool to help others.

Countless doctors, nurses, and medical experts give their hearts and souls to the profession and probably don't get the rewards they deserve. It took Denise's death to fully appreciate the value of those great doctors and to experience how much bad doctors can take from us.

We may never have the type of documentation necessary for accountability. But I will go through my life knowing that this could and should have been prevented. I will live the rest of my time on Earth painfully aware that when Denise needed all of us, we didn't listen to her.

Chapter 14

Nine-Month Attachments

As I continued to battle the demons in my head, I worked toward a better life. I wished I could fast forward to years ahead to move past some of the pain. I never wanted this lonely life. As much anger as I had toward the medical community and God, I recognized that I could only control myself. I would do whatever I could to take care of the life I now was being forced to live.

I remained grateful for the students who worked hard in my classroom. I desired to be as dedicated a teacher as they were as students. As long as they were learning and achieving, I was happy to provide an easy-going approach. Of course, I could always be the teacher who gets firm when things got out of hand. I understood the value of getting the students to do what was necessary.

When students who came to my class daily gave me their very best, I in turn felt obligated to give them mine. My students know that, if they come to class ready to learn, I will do everything in my power to keep the group progressing while having some fun. This classroom philosophy enabled me to develop good relationships with parents and students. Even before Denise's passing, I had structures in place. When everything went wrong, I still had those students who did their utmost to learn. In a lot of ways, those relationships were the only ones I maintained on a daily basis. I valued the structure and enjoyment of teaching. I doubt that many of those students whom I had the opportunity to teach will ever know what they truly did for me. They made me feel valued and helped me more than I could ever have imagined as I grieved.

I often went to the gym or did some kind of exercise at home regularly. I continued to wake up at 5:30 a.m. each day and tried my best to deal with my stress before school. I struggled to eliminate as much of the pressure I was feeling as I could, but painful thoughts permeated my mind. Although there was little escape from my feelings, exercise brought a welcome release, and I was happy I could use it as therapy while I attempted to get my body back into a stronger, healthier state.

Thanks to the structures I built for my life, I was making gains. Even so, with the exception of grocery shopping on Fridays and going to Bill and Judy's for pizza, I continued to stay very much to myself most of the time. I would occasionally break out of my routine, but I have always valued structure, and this tragedy just reinforced that.

Little by little over time, I built toward overcoming another hurdle. I wanted someday to be able to wean myself off the sleep medication. From the moment I started taking sleeping pills, I knew there would come a time when I would have to work to stop. Denise wouldn't have wanted me to live with the depression and sleep medication, so from the beginning I tried not to let taking them develop into an addiction. My goal was to keep myself as healthy as possible physically, emotionally, and psychologically. Dependence on sleep medication did not fit with that aspiration.

I had managed to stay alive and remain in the moment as much as possible. When the time came to wean off the sleep meds, I had already built the extreme structure in myself necessary to make the attempt. Maintain the daily routines of rising and going to bed early would give me a much better chance at removing the support of the medication.

When I felt that I was ready, I succeeded in giving up those pills. I was proud of how well I did. Although I knew I might need them on occasion at some point, getting myself off them was a major step in the right direction.

Because I got up early and I gave 100% to my students, I tended to wear down by the afternoon. I quickly learned that I would need some caffeine to keep me going. I've never been much of a coffee drinker, and I had tried for a while to avoid drinking soda, but my body needed something to keep me going at the level I wanted to perform. I started bringing two-liter bottles of Diet Coke to work so I could have one cup in the afternoon. Although I intended to let go of this habit as soon as I could, for the time being I figured soda was probably my best option to get through the afternoon.

Soon after Denise's death, I decided I wouldn't drink alcohol for fear of where it would lead me. During the week of the funeral, while spending time with relatives, I tried a sip of liquor that Bill and Judy had, but, apart from that one drink, I didn't touch alcohol. I had a few beers in the fridge and happily gave those away.

Denise and I had a full wine rack. I kept a lot of those bottles because many of them represented places we had been and fun times we shared. I knew alcohol was a slippery slope into deeper depression, so I continued to stay away from it.

Since I had never really been a drug user, I was always more concerned about the drugs that were prescribed to me, and, now that I was off my sleep meds, I was happy to be as healthy as I could be, all things considered.

Because of the mounting number of things I was being asked to handle single-handedly, I got into a routine of taking care of one small task every day after school. Every weekend I had a list of items to get done. I had done this while Denise was still alive. She used to make fun of me, saying, "Now you can cross it off your list." Then she would famously roll her eyes.

On top of my weekend agenda, I started a weekday to-do list. Every day I had something lined up for after school. There were days I needed to get home and make a phone call; on other days I would buy gas. Sometimes I needed to drop by the bank or visit Target to pick up a few things.

The benefit of my weekday after-school itinerary was that it freed my Saturdays and Sundays for more rest. I appreciated spending time on the couch where I could relax and recover in order to get my body ready for the week ahead.

During the school week I taught, performed my one task each evening, and then came home to eat leftovers for dinner. Since I was the only one in the house, often I used the weekends to prepare meals for the week ahead. I didn't have enough energy to cook by the time I got home on a workday.

This routine seemed to work for me. After I arrived home, usually I changed my clothes, sorted the mail, made my sandwich for the next day, ate dinner, cleaned afterward, and then watched TV until about 8:30 p.m. I was pretty used to the routine, which helped me get myself back together a lot. I still didn't talk to too many people and actually kept my phone off for most of the evening. I occasionally texted people, but rarely did I talk much on the phone at night. I just did my best to pass the time and give my body enough rest to face another tomorrow in this sad new normal I was developing.

I usually fell asleep pretty quickly due to my routines. After relaxing on the sofa, I brushed my teeth and wrote or typed my nightly letter to Denise before crawling into bed. I finished my night by reading for a half hour. This routine helped me immeasurably to regain balance amidst the loneliness and sadness.

I tried to keep my mind busy on various projects. Looking back on the 5K, I considered how well it went and what we could implement so that the next year's event would be better. Working on my Lego dream house kept my brain engaged with designing, ordering individual pieces, and assembling the set. I had been given a couple of podcasts that were beneficial to listen to and supported my need to keep my mind active with healthy thoughts. Also, I spent hours decompressing, mulling over things people had said and contemplating challenges that were approaching, including the nine-month anniversary of Denise's passing.

After the six-month mark, I worried about what the next quarter year point had in store. So many of my routines still centered around honoring Denise's memory and staying connected to her. I knew I would need to pull back on some of those activities. I had done a great job of preserving her legacy as I released the grief as much as I could.

I had made it through three-quarters of a year without the woman I loved. The sense of loss remained intense. I was still here but I was a shell of the man I was before my life became so damaged. At the six-month point, I had started typing our love story, the chronicle of our years together. I was almost finished with that, but I still couldn't fathom letting go of this ritual that connected me to Denise at the end of each day. I decided that after I completed the love story, ending with the last night we were together, I would type all of my nightly reflections as well. I still wasn't ready to step away from Denise and needed to have something in place to fill that void. I opted to type three of those reflections each evening. It would allow me to spend the last part of my night before bed focused on Denise.

Transitioning from writing about our final night together to the first night after my world was rocked brought an awakening I wasn't prepared for. As I typed, the darkness of those first few days seemed overwhelming. Even so, it acted as a kind of therapy, revealing how far I had progressed in such a short period. I still felt as if the tragedy had just happened. At the same time, it seemed I had lived much more than nine months during that span. It was a weird feeling as I sat and typed those dark memories. It was heart wrenching that I needed to tell this story, but I was relieved I was able to find the words.

For nine months I had books and biographies about grief every night as a means of coping. Some were really helpful and others not so much. I felt it was time to get back to some other forms of reading, but I had to figure out what kinds of books

I could read. I had found crime thrillers and legal fiction so interesting before this happened. Not anymore.

I ended up finding a couple of books that dealt with funny or happy themes. The first book I read was about a group of MIT students who went to Las Vegas and had a bunch of fun counting cards. I needed these light-hearted stories, which stayed so much away from dark subjects, to reintegrate back into the world of reading that I had always enjoyed.

When the question of the wedding ring came up again, I thought I would be able to take it off but still wasn't ready. I knew I would have to remove it at some point, but a large part of me felt so saddened by the thought. This challenge was a monster I would face sometime in the future. I knew I was no longer married. I realized I hadn't seen my beautiful wife in nine months. But the thought of being ready to separate myself from Denise was still too overwhelming. I decided I would wait until the one-year mark. I might have to force myself to remove the ring then. I still wasn't ready to cross that hurdle.

All of these difficulties seemed small compared to something I really didn't want to do. For as long as I knew Denise, there was one aspect of her that I loved over everything, and that was her smile. I had loved that smile since the first time I saw it. While she was alive, I craved those moments when I got her to smile. Her inner light beamed through that beautiful smile. In every photo of us, the wonder of her smile shone.

I had missed that human smile for nine months. During that time, I had watched the film that Dawn and Brian made every week to relive the good times we had shared and hold in my heart the caring and wonderful person Denise was.

I used that film to retrain my brain so that, instead of reliving the horror of her loss and the image of her lifeless body, I could vividly recall her life and all those precious moments we shared. I cried so many times sitting by her niche on Sunday mornings, even when I thought I couldn't possibly have any more tears. Then I came home after church, put on the film, and watched only to realize how many tears I still had to shed.

Both of my parents found it difficult to watch the film with me when they stayed at the house. I understood how hard it was. Nonetheless, every Sunday after church I came home to view that video. Although it hurt to do so, I always wanted to remember Denise for what she was in life rather than the devastation of her death.

I decided to move away from replaying the video at the nine-month point. This was not something I wanted to do, but I knew it would be another step in the direction of healing.

Two weeks before the nine-month mark, I stood in church, listening to the congregation sing some joyous song that probably uplifted everyone in the sanctuary apart from Bill, Judy, and me. I realized at that moment that the three-quarters of a year date would fall on a Sunday. I instantly started to cry, feeling the weight of what I had approaching. I stood there with tears running down my face, recognizing that in a couple weeks I would leave church after visiting the niche only to go home and view the video for the last weekly time. It was tough to comprehend. Long ago I gave up trying to wipe my tears away in public. I wanted people to see who I really was and the tears revealed the real me.

The week before the date arrived, I continued to cry during the singing at church, knowing that very soon I would be letting go of something I didn't want to pull away from. I understood that it was a step in the right direction, but that didn't alter my feelings.

The difficulty of marking three-quarters of a year came as expected. I still felt sick that this beautiful woman no longer stood beside me with our babies. It was all so sad. My heart ached through the church service, and sitting out at the niche continued to be gut-wrenching. Going home alone was awful too.

I put on the video and sat through what seemed like a four-hour production rather than a thirty-minute film. Every picture touched me. The fact that I wouldn't be watching this next week seemed unreal. I hated making those necessary steps to move on with a life that was still unknown to me. I didn't want any of this. But I was willing to meet those moments head on.

As the final scenes played, the understanding that this was just another step I had to take sank in. I was forced to look at the fact that Denise was never coming back. This life was never meant to give me its very best. This loss was wrong on so many levels. The last picture, one of our Christmas card photos, seemed so sad. Watching that 30 minutes of video destroyed me inside, knowing I had to let it go.

Denise was so beautiful. Every photograph showed that this world was a much better one with her in it. The worst of the world ended something so wonderful in a horrific way. As I removed the video from the player, the pain overwhelmed me. But Denise wouldn't have wanted to see me fall into the darkness. She made me into the person I was, and, because of that, I knew I had to set aside this weekly ritual. The video would be there on the shelf when those moments came to relive the love we shared. But I couldn't watch it with the same consistency and still move forward.

I wondered how I would spend the time every Sunday. I decided to visit the gym during that time frame to release my anxiety and work out all my emptiness, knowing what those 30 minutes represented.

I had made it through another hurdle on my way to proving I could survive. I wasn't proud of all my choices or of how I continued to handle everything. However, I was pleased that I was still alive, and I think Denise would have been proud of me for the strides I had made. I had put support in place, removing some of it gradually as I was able. I knew I wasn't ready to take off the ring. That sad day would come. But I would never again see the person I loved nor would I experience and share the joy that was ours. Remembering that life evoked pure beauty as well as pure sadness. I faced the reality of living in the moment, and the more moments you live, the more life you have. I would continue the good fight even as I still struggled. I continued to live in sorrow, wanting so much to have the life I really thought Denise and I were meant to share.

Chapter 15

Empty and Alone

When tragedies occur, early on there is so much support and it is so overwhelming. Looking back on how I managed that first week, I think the main reason I was able to keep myself together was the huge amount of support we received. So many people let us know they cared about the whole family. The enormity of our tragedy failed to sink in fully as a result of being in shock and having the community come to our aid. I wasn't able to fully understand what Denise's passing meant at the time. I just knew I wanted to write a speech worthy of her life for the funeral and read it on the last day I would see her.

In the shock of grief when you are buoyed by so many people coming forward to help, you feel a kind of stamina that begins to diminish afterward. I knew that I would need people with me for a long time. During my talk to my school, I mentioned how this tragedy would remain with me. While others would go back to their lives, I would need many of the people to continue the outpouring of kindness.

The reality of my situation was the loss of three lives. Beyond that though, I lost the life I was all supposed to have. The passing of Denise and those babies was bad enough, but I soon realized that everything I had built toward was gone. The dream of a future with my wife and children had died too. I didn't know what to do and how to fully navigate the depth of my pain.

I was fortunate my parents could stay with me for most of the remainder of the first school year. January was a cruel month for a number of reasons. I watched the house transform from a home for Denise and me and our babies to a place where my life had to continue without them. Luckily Dawn and Judy took care of cleaning the nursery and Denise's clothes. Yet, I still had to come home to that sad, empty house every day.

I experienced a sense of hollowness in January, but there were still enough tasks to keep me busy, to occupy my troubled thoughts. Seeing the nursery become just a guestroom was deeply painful for me. The life Denise and I had worked so hard to build was literally being taken apart. One day her closet was full of clothes and the next day no trace remained of her there. All good things do come to an end, but this was an end for which I was totally unprepared.

As the house transformed, I was grateful to have Dad return and stay with me for as long as he did. His help and kindness gave me strength for what I had to do. Words cannot describe how much better it was to drive home knowing someone was at the house. Dad was really good for me on an emotional and psychological level. In January, it was really hard coming home to the empty house. Nonetheless, I knew there would come a time when Dad would visit again; all I had to do was hold on until his next trip.

Later, in the summer, when Dad headed home after helping a huge amount with the race, I had difficulty coping. I was alone much of the time. I drove home to an empty house to sleep in an empty bed. The next day I would wake up in that empty bed and repeat the cycle.

I lived the single life for a long time before meeting Denise. I had been an only child and, up until Denise and I moved in together, I was fine just being by myself. Still, now that I was dealing with this massive hole in my heart and the hollowness that I felt and that the house represented, I struggled to keep myself upbeat. I dealt with depression but never wanted to take any medication. My feelings weren't as raw as they once had been, but I hated what my life had morphed into. I saw no way to break out of this defeat and loneliness.

By this point everyone had gotten back to their lives. The intense emotions people experienced when they found out what happened had worn off. I became an afterthought. I was just stuck in this daily depression. I wanted the lives others had, but instead I had no life. The one I was prepared for was never going to happen. I was completely heartbroken. These feelings weighed heavily on me. It was a challenging situation and one I wished no one to ever understand. I wouldn't wish these circumstances and this grief on anyone.

Since people had gotten back to their lives, I tried to pretend everything was going to be okay. I would be all right just suffering through this strange new world, but I wasn't doing well. During those empty months alone, I felt a level of sadness that was sometimes too overwhelming to really reflect on.

When everything happened and the school stepped up to bring me dinners, that amazing gesture gave me something to look forward to at night. I conversed with my parents by phone about who was coming over and how I knew them. My parents were trading on-and-off weeks to spend time with me. Now that the dinners were no longer coming, and my parents were back home, it was just me.

Two of Denise's friends, Kelly and Gus, decided to step up and ask if they could come sit with me a couple of times a month. After I agreed they traded visits, sitting with me and talking.

Most of us probably take for granted how nice it is to arrive home at the end of the day and have someone there to just talk about things. When it is all gone, it's a wretched feeling.

Apart from my students and Mr. Bob, I didn't talk much after Denise's passing. As a result, I developed bad habits and often spent most of the time talking rather than listening. I spoke so little with people outside of the classroom that I lost the art of conversation. I ended up often controlling the discussion because I rarely had time to share my feelings out loud to others. Kelly and Gus recognized how difficult my life had become; their empathy and understanding helped me.

The best card I received during that first Christmas was from a co-worker who wrote, "Hopefully this card will make your Christmas a little less shitty." It was one of the few cards that made me smile.

I really wished to feel less alone, but, no matter where I went, no matter what I did, at the end of the day I still returned to an empty house. I could do nothing to change that fact. This was my life. As much as I didn't want to live in it, I had no choice.

Kelly and Gus were really good for me, but, like all good things, their bimonthly visits came to an end. Although it pained me, they needed to return to their lives. To be honest, Kelly and Gus had been with me since day one. They fully understood where I was and the fact that it was going to take a number of months or even years to get back to where I used to be if I ever could. They wanted to be with me, and I greatly appreciated the outpouring of love and support they gave.

A number of other friends whom Denise really cared for and was close to honestly didn't reach out to me much if at all. People had their own lives and, while I understood that, I still had to figure out how to live my life. I never felt I needed to tell people how bad this tragedy was for me. Perhaps if I had, I would have received more support. Rather than remind them of all I had lost, I let them go about their own lives.

People deal with grief in their own way. Much of my grief stemmed from the fact that my daily structure was centered around Denise. I struggled with the idea that people had to get back to their own lives. I felt they were moving on without me. It was a hard notion for me to grasp.

Many of the issues I was dealing with related to the ways I was handling everything. I didn't let many people know how depressed I really was. As a result, people who would have gone out of their way to continue to support me didn't. It was a challenge for me to reach out to people. I didn't like calling people to let them know I wasn't doing well. Consequently, Mr. Bob, Bill and Judy, and my parents were really about the only people who knew the state I was in. Most people were probably too afraid to ask how I was holding up.

I have always prided myself on not being selfish; maybe I should have been more selfish. I just wanted other people to be happy, so during those months I didn't reach out to let others know how hard life was or to express the things I needed to get me through those lonely evenings. I didn't want my diluted view of the world to infect others, so I further isolated myself at the single worst time to do so.

I wanted our friends to get back to their wonderful lives, but I didn't want to deal with the fact that they had done so. I was heartbroken.

Although I didn't believe I was forgotten, I thought I was someone who made people feel sad. Years ago I had a really good friend who was in the military and got deployed. I knew how hard it was for him to be away from his wife and daughter, and I wanted to do something to help. I wrote to him every week. I wanted to make sure he knew that even though I didn't see him daily I was thinking about him. When he came home, he told me he had learned who his real friends were and who would always be there for him while he was away.

I felt a lot of the emotions he had during his deployment, just in a much different situation. People at work continued to be concerned for me but they saw how upbeat I was because of how I felt working with those students. To the students' credit, I was cheerful in the classroom, because the more they worked, the more fun we could all have. I was lucky that I was in that environment. Nevertheless, come the end of the day, I would be going home to a place that was empty.

I have never enjoyed phone conversations, so many of the discussions I found myself having came in the form of text messages. I highly valued getting a text or a card. I felt grateful for the people who continued to remember that I was in pain.

How do you text someone to tell them you hate your life so much? There were a lot of people who cared about me. Sadly, they had no idea about my pain because I didn't let others know. I couldn't bring myself to inflict my sadness on them. I didn't want to bring a cloud of darkness into other people's light. Choosing not to reach out made my grieving harder.

I struggled with vacations because the thought of coming home was always challenging. Why build a time of happiness only to have it end and have to return to the reality of my situation? Often I've found that the hardest falls are the ones from the greatest heights.

In September, Denise's family was planning a trip to Disney and had asked me to go with them. The invitation was a really nice gesture. Although we all knew that so much had changed, we seemed to continue to get along really well when we were together.

I knew this was their trip, and I was just along for the ride. They didn't mind that, of course, and were happy I was coming, but internally I struggled with feeling like an outsider.

Denise and I had spent many of our work breaks joining her family on trips to Disney. Before she passed, we had bought tickets so that we could go. But because of her pregnancy, we were happy we could save those tickets for a more entertaining trip with those wonderful twins.

With Denise's passing, I still had the tickets and figured she would want me to go. I battled internally about what to do with the other ticket, Denise's ticket. A part of me didn't feel right going to Disney on two separate occasions because of her passing. I realized the best way to handle the situation was to explain to Disney what had happened and see if they could do something to help another family. Unfortunately, Disney was not able to do this for me. I felt really bad for the customer service guy who had to tell me they weren't able to take back the tickets as tears streamed from my eyes. The best I could do was randomly give them to a family.

The first family I saw, standing right next to the customer service desk, was astonished that I offered them those free days to Disney; they honestly didn't know what to make of the situation. I told them there was a five-day park hopper on the card that I wasn't going to use, and I wanted it to go to some family who could enjoy it. I explained that the customer service representative, who was still at the counter watching this exchange, would vouch for it being legit. They offered me money but I told them I just wanted them to have a good time even if it wasn't on this trip and tried to leave before I began crying again in public.

I made it out the doors before I started weeping and caught up with Bill and Judy. I shared what happened with them; they understood and knew the situation was painful for me.

A minute or two later, I felt a tapping on my shoulder. It was the family I had given the tickets to. The customer service gentleman had told them the reason I wanted to find a good home for the tickets. They explained to me that they had another daughter at home, in addition to the one who was with them on this trip, whom they would take to Disney with the ticket at a later time.

I knew that's what Denise would have wanted. I hugged the wife to thank her for her understanding. It was a really hard moment. In this place that is built on cheerful memories, where Denise and I had shared joyful times, the sadness and happiness intermingled within my heart.

The rest of the trip was really good. We all had a pleasant time. Still, even joyful moments were shrouded by the underlying awareness of what my life would be once I returned home. When I was with Denise's family, I was an add-on to their vacation. They didn't view my presence like that, and I'm sure they were happy I came along, but this was my internal viewpoint.

Spending the vacation with Bill and Judy and the family brought us all closer. However, the highs from being on a vacation to the lows of walking back into the house alone were challenging. The drop off after a high can cause greater pain than continuing to live in the daily grind of depression.

Even so, that daily despair was a dreadful state. I hated the life I was being forced to live without Denise, without our family. Knowing this was the only life I was allowed to live now, I determined to suffer through the difficult moments.

I continued to listen to my podcasts about sports and other topics to keep my brain engaged. I was always afraid my lack of regular human connection with people my own age would cause my mental state to deteriorate. I tried not let the emptiness and loneliness I felt have any long-lasting, devastating effects. Still, I was in a really bad place for most of the year.

Keeping up the house, cooking, and cleaning kept me busy. Finding the time to mow the lawn and still relax enough proved challenging. As long as I kept my extreme structure, I could stay ahead of the housework and daily tasks that I needed to do as I dealt with the sad reality of living by myself.

Exercising provided a big release for me, and I continued to talk with Mr. Bob. I kept up with my Lego projects and read some books that kept me upbeat. Grocery shopping remained part of my Friday evening routine. I maintained this regimented existence to better help with the reality of the situation. However, because I had so many projects and things I needed to accomplish to keep my brain occupied, I found little time for socializing when the opportunity presented itself.

I had spent so many hours dedicated to putting on the 5K race that once it was over I fell right back into my everyday struggle. Even when friends reached out and asked me to visit, I felt that I wouldn't be able to get everything done if I spent the time with them. I was concerned that if I did get out of the house, I would fall behind in my tasks. I had put myself in a really odd, catch-22 position. I felt I couldn't break out of the structure I had created to deal with the loneliness. Even when I had opportunities to relieve my solitude, I wasn't able to relinquish the very routines I built to help me through the aloneness. I ended up forming a tough situation. But it was a far better alternative than not staying busy.

I knew I needed to keep my mind occupied to deal with how sad and dark my life was; yet in doing so I made my circumstances worse. I rigorously maintained my routine. I lined things up a week in advance to be able to prepare for accomplishing my tasks. When people would ask me to come for dinner, often I wasn't able to break free of the structure I had put in place to deal with what was going in my head and heart.

I found it was best to combine activities I already had planned, such as watching a sporting event, which doubled as my relaxation time, with getting together with a friend if they would watch too. This was how I was able to walk the fine line between trying to be social and still fulfilling all my tasks.

Luckily, I had an opportunity arise to tutor a former student, and I was asked to help coach a youth boys' basketball team. These were planned activities I could work into my schedule that would provide an opportunity for social interaction. The demons inside of my head and the emptiness of my heart remained, but I tried to live as best I could in this world that was never meant for giving me its best.

I worked diligently to remain busy as a means of dealing with the sadness. My brain required distractions and respite from the misery. I still often wept when I was in the shower because it was about the only time I wasn't able to distract myself.

The kindness of friends and family who cared for me had gotten me this far, but their own lives needed to continue, and I didn't want to reach out to them to let them know how desperately I needed their help.

If a tree falls in the forest, does anyone hear it? I often have pondered that question. I thought of the comparison between myself and the fallen tree. Since I didn't tell people how I was holding up, they never knew. They may have assumed that my life was terrible, and it very much was. Most of those horrible moments happened at the house where I lived. Because no one was there with me, no one really knew nor could they help. I thought to myself, *If no one knows how bad off I am, if I don't tell anyone, no one will really understand.*

I was alone and there wasn't much that could be done about that. The house was now my house. None of the smiling pictures that hung on the walls could bring back the life I thought I was going to lead. It was my job to suffer through these moments and hope that my sadness, anger, and emptiness didn't rob others of the joy in their lives.

Even in the midst of my loneliness, I hoped there were others who had returned to lives of joy. There wasn't much anyone could do to change my life at this point. I had to find my way and learn to travel the path of loss. I internalized a lot of my feelings to avoid inflicting my sorrow on those around me. Apart from Mr. Bob and my parents, no one truly saw the real me.

I felt empty and alone. I lived in a house that was perfect for four. I was trying to wait until all the bad got better and hope that when I came out of this, I could still see the good. I had isolated myself both for my own protection as well as other people's happiness. For those souls who continued to think of me and the daily struggle I was going through, I will never forget how much their caring meant to me even on those ordinary days, not only on the significant ones. I seemed to need the most help on those *everydays*.

The days all ran together and were all sad. My life was an empty pit that I was scratching and clawing to get out of.

I rested in the house. I lived in the house. And sooner or later I would have to figure out how I was going to be able to function as a man so broken and beaten down. I knew that soon the time would come when I had to remove a ring that I never wanted to take off. Only then to continue to come home to a house that was so empty and a heart that was so broken and to attempt to live through each day only to wake up in that same world the next day and do it all over again.

Chapter 16

One-Year Anniversary

Although my life continued to be difficult, I prepared myself for some days more than others. From the beginning, when my emotions felt overwhelming, I just tried to make it to the 23rd of every month. Then I set goals to endure until the six-month mark and to reach the nine-month point. After managing up to that time, I struggled those first couple of weeks after not watching the film. Yet, thanks to spending that period on Sunday afternoons at the gym, I got used to not watching the film then and was able to better handle myself. The next hurdle would come at the one-year anniversary of my broken heart.

I both anticipated and feared that day. October 23, 2017, was going to fall on a Monday, and I worried the entire weekend leading up to the date.

That morning I woke up to the sound of my alarm clock after a reasonable night of sleep. I turned off the alarm and promptly got moving. I had planned for the worst and hoped for the best. The ideal thing to do was to stay busy from the moment I awakened. I quickly was out the door, driving to the gym, which seemed to be my getaway spot when I needed to remove myself from the house and what it represented.

After the gym, the sadness over took me in the shower. I got out as soon as I could to seek distraction, in this case my iPod. I was able to get to work a little earlier than usual, which was understandable because this was not a day to stop moving.

I had previously spoken with Mrs. Lanane, one of the great co-workers who helped me *dry up the well* by visiting her office and talking. I hadn't done that much in a while, but there were still days when I benefited greatly from the release of emotions and tears. I was aware the anniversary of Denise's passing would intensify my emotions, so I made advance arrangements to help me survive the day. Mrs. Lanane and I had discussed whether or not I wanted to take the day off and what I had planned. I tried to prepare myself as best I could for the arrival of that anniversary. Mrs. Lanane was understanding and kind. We talked about how we felt the day would go. We both knew that it was going to be bad and that was the truth of the situation.

I cried and discussed the anticipation of how I would handle the day up until the bell rang, and then I was off to my classroom for my eight-hour distraction. As I walked to class, I knew that this would be a day of reflection, of remembering all that Denise had brought to my life. I had lived a year without her. I hated what my life had become, but, as I walked to class, I realized just being alive was a sad victory in itself. I believed Denise was proud of me for getting through the saddest year of my life.

My time at school went smoothly. I was surprised as to how well I handled the workday considering the sad agenda I had planned for after school. I imagined I would start to break down walking out at the end of the day, but surprisingly the aftereffects of teaching and staying busy buoyed me. I started to really feel the weight of my emotions while standing in line for the bank teller. There was a new guy working, one who didn't know my sad story. He helped me deposit the house insurance check I had received after a large hail storm in early September damaged the roof beyond repair. As he was preparing my check, he sensed that my emotions were about to get the best of me. After he completed the transaction, I asked to get into my safety deposit box.

He went and got the paperwork and I followed him to where all the boxes were kept. He drew out my box and I told him I would need the privacy room that is kept for people with safety deposit boxes. I went in, shut the door, and started to break down. Knowing what I was there to do, I couldn't hold back the tears. I opened the box and looked at its contents. Denise's Pandora charm bracelet held each of the individual charms that I had bought for her on trips I took since her passing. I then pulled out the box that held her engagement ring and opened it. As I held it in my hand, I sobbed.

I hated that moment. I wished with all my being that this wasn't my life. I looked at her engagement ring and then touched her wedding ring which I had continued to wear on a chain every day. Reluctantly, I gazed down at my own wedding ring and, with a deep breath, pulled it off my finger. I placed it around her engagement ring and, holding them both, I let the tears come. It was such a sad moment, my moment. I never imagined the kind of pain I had felt during that lonely, miserable year. I wished so much that her passing and all of this pain had never happened. Through the blur of tears, I looked at the two rings together and knew nothing would ever be the same.

It took me a few moments to collect myself. But, finally, I kissed the rings, placed them back in the case, and then closed the safety deposit box. The teller helped me return it safely to its slot, and I thanked him for his help and headed home. I was overwhelmed as I walked out of the bank—more depressed than ever. I felt heartbroken as I drove home realizing more tears would fall that evening.

When I got home, I ended up talking to a law firm about the aftermath of Denise's death and my moral obligation to make certain I did my part to ensure this never happened again. If it did, I could not live with myself unless I had done everything possible to prevent it. After talking with the attorney, I changed my clothes and got ready to leave the house.

I needed to visit the niche. Like so many other special days, this time would be spent at the columbarium. Since I had planned to go to her resting place, I had prepared my dinner the previous day to take with me. By the time I arrived at the church, a light rain was falling, so I angled my car to look over at the columbarium while I ate my meal in the car.

I knew that I was going to post something to Facebook. Seeing as how I rarely post, I always want to share something meaningful. Although I had done month-by-month postings, my last one was at the nine-month mark. I knew which picture I would share for the longest time. It was a photo that was taken of Denise and me as we laughed outside of our brand-new house on the day we closed. She was so happy in the moment and so precious.

I uploaded the picture to Facebook and continued to eat. After I finished, I got out of the car, grabbed my folding chair, and walked over to the niche. The rain had cleared and I sat there as I had done so many times before and just cried.

I sat there until after sunset. I talked to her and to our kids and reflected on what that day was, how it was never supposed to like this. It was too sad to be real. If some fiction writer were making up a story, they couldn't have written a sadder ending than we had.

I stayed at her niche until dark, trying to take in the moment, realizing a full year had passed from that terrible day when everything became wrong. We were robbed of the life we should have had, and now I was walking away to go home to an empty house. As I drove home in the darkness, the gloom of night reflected the state of my life.

When I got home, I had one more task; it wasn't going to be as difficult as removing my ring, but it would still be hard.

I pulled out the film that was created for the viewing, the one I had watched so many times during the first nine months, put it in to play, and prepared myself for more crying.

I was surprised at the effect of watching the movie had on me that evening. Although emotion still welled with me, I didn't cry as much as I imagined I would. I saw the photos and remembered how beautiful and full of life Denise was. Brian did a wonderful job of adding the music to the video.

The third song was always my favorite as well as the hardest to hear. I arrived at the part of the film that showed the photos from our last trip to Florida when we had visited a former co-worker at her house in The Villages. I knew by heart what came next. The picture that followed always brought the deepest sadness. There she stood in the old house. She was in her first trimester, glowing with love and joy. Every time that picture appeared, I could not contain the sorrow.

I would have thought the pictures of her closer to her due date would have had the most effect on me, but for some reason it was that shot taken during the first trimester. I was lying down as I watched the video and instantly felt the emotion build to overflowing. I had always known where that snapshot was in the video, and often my anxiety would build up as that place in the film neared. Then when I saw that picture I would cry out. The same thing happened during this viewing. Like so many other times, I tried to pull myself together quickly so I didn't miss any of the other beautiful moments captured on camera, all of which revealed the wonder that was Denise. Such sadness and emptiness ruled my world now. I wished that kind of pain on nobody.

At the conclusion of the movie, I called Dad and talked to him. It was about 8:00 p.m. by this time, and normally I would be relaxing until about 8:30 when I started to get ready for bed. However, that evening I talked to him past 8:30 because I needed to. We discussed my day, how sad it was, and how the worst part was taking off the ring. Dad and I had previously conversed about whether or not I needed to remove the ring. I knew I had to because Denise was no longer living. I truly never wanted to take it off but believed it was a necessary step. Dad understood. After talking with him, I felt better. So many emotions had been building since I left school that the release was important. It felt really good to talk to Dad.

I received a wonderful outpouring of love that day both before I posted the picture on Facebook as well as after. People showed me compassion, which I deeply appreciated, but I remained reserved; I knew all of this love and support was only a temporary Band-Aid that would be gone within a few days. People had their own lives to live, so I understood that, no matter how many people gave me strength that day, tomorrow, even though it wouldn't be as difficult, was still going to be another empty, lonely day only without the outpouring of encouragement. I had been down this road enough that year to realize this truth. Still, I valued everyone's kindness on the one-year anniversary. I told myself that everyday wasn't going to be as difficult even though I still lived in my depression.

I read many of the comments people wrote in response to my Facebook post and felt happy they cared. When I signed out of Facebook that evening, I deleted the app on my phone. After Denise's passing, I found it difficult to look at Facebook. I would get so angry at seeing what others thought were important issues. My heart-filled posts were often drowned out by people posting about food and other things that didn't compare to what I was dealing with.

Most importantly, I felt jealous of the pictures people posted of their happy lives. I couldn't handle seeing happy families going on vacations, knowing that this was something that I would never be able to do with Denise and those kids. Often I scanned my Facebook feed in case something important was posted, but after a while I just couldn't take it anymore. I appreciated that Facebook had helped me when the sadness was at its worst in the beginning, but at this point it only seemed to amplify my struggle.

That night of the one-year anniversary, I heard from a couple of people who rarely reached out. I found it challenging to deal with them because I expected to hear more from them during the year. I never wanted to be the person to tell others they had let me down by forgetting about my daily battle to continue living.

One of the things people often asked me was what they could do for me. The answer was simple: they could get in touch, send me a text, and let me know that they were thinking of me.

I really struggled to make my life better. In the midst of that, letting people know they had let me down was hard to do. But that night I expressed my disappointment to one of Denise's friends. I told her that if she thought of me all the time, then she shouldn't wait four months to let me know.

Every day was hard, and yes, the one-year anniversary was especially so even though I was prepared for it. The sad reality was that the rest of the week was still going to be painful. The difference was that I wasn't building up for those days, planning how to handle them. Instead I just continued living in those incredibly agonizing moments.

The reality was that today people remembered Denise and thought about what I was living through. Sadly, the more days that passed, the more people would get back to their lives. If I were in their shoes, I may very well have done the same thing; I'm not trying to say that people weren't there for me; however, only some were. When every day is challenging, it's really difficult to have one day that you hear from so many only to have no one reach out three days later.

If anyone I know goes through something like this, I will know firsthand how important it is to connect with that person. I just hoped with all of my heart that no one else ever suffered like this. I couldn't imagine how other people dealt with the overwhelming amount of pain that I had.

I still had so many unanswered questions. As bad as this life was at the moment, I appreciated the people who cared and was thankful I had made it through what will probably be the worst year of my life. I wasn't a better person for it, but I had survived. I was profoundly changed and only time would tell how much. The reality was that I was here and I was still surviving.

Chapter 17

The Kids' First Birthday

Making it through the one-year anniversary was a step in the right direction. It was a sorrowful day but one that I was proud I had survived. Still, countless more tough days lay ahead. I had to face the most intense issues at that point. Nonetheless, every day brought the challenges that went into continuing to try to live in this world.

People got back to their lives and I fell quickly back into my normal routine. The following weekend I did hear from a friend who forgot to text me on the Monday anniversary of her passing. I told her I appreciated her forgetting because

I had heard from many people on Monday, but by Saturday everyone had gotten back to their lives. I was thankful for a gesture of support on one of those "every days." She was glad her mistake made me feel good.

With the one-year anniversary past, I was feeling anxious for something that was coming up very shortly. The last day of October, Halloween, was going to be difficult for a variety of reasons. I decided the previous year to do something that would acknowledge those two precious twins who passed away with Denise. I wanted to dedicate Denise's passing date to her alone, so I decided I would always remember the twins on Halloween, which was the date Denise's C-section had been scheduled. If everything had gone well, the doctors would have delivered those babies on October 31, and our family would be whole. Since, sadly, that was not the case, instead I put some activities in place, things to always remember the kids. I selected activities I thought Denise and I would have done with those kids to celebrate their birthday.

The year before Bill, Judy, Dad, and I walked around one of the local parks and then went for ice cream. I felt I could repeat these every year to remind me of the kids. That first Halloween our loss was still so fresh. Since I was still out of school, we spent the time together that day sharing pastimes that Denise and I might have enjoyed with our children. Now that I was working, it could be a little more challenging. I decided earlier in the month I would go ahead and take the day off. That way I would have time to get to the park and get ice cream before the trick-or-treaters showed up at my door. Last year I had passed out candy with Dad and the police investigator, Ryan, who was nice enough to visit with us.

I was lucky enough to find a substitute teacher and get the time off. I had considered taking Denise's passing date off from work, but I believed she would have wanted to me do something to commemorate our children who meant so much to her. She cherished family, so I felt certain she would want me to choose pastimes we could spend together.

Since I had the day off, I tried again to set up a couple of appointments. My personal doctor, whom I wanted to see, was unavailable that day, so I thought long and hard about the other appointment and decided to make the call.

One morning before school started, I called the OB/GYN Denise saw. I asked for the office manager and was forwarded to his phone. Luckily for both of us, he wasn't at his desk, so I left a message asking to have a meeting with them. I was well aware of the current issues we all faced and mentioned that I understood if they would be unable to take the meeting, but I felt I needed to ask. I let them know if they wanted to bring their lawyers I had no issues with that.

I was glad I left a message because I would have felt bad for the office manager if he picked up the phone completely unprepared for the uncomfortable request I had. I left my message and moved on. I figured that once the office manager heard it he would reach out to their law department to try to figure out what their availability was. It took a couple of days, but the office manager left a message letting me know that he and the doctor who was the last one at the firm to see Denise, would meet me on October 31, the date that would have been the twins' birthday.

I knew that my request had put them in an uncomfortable position. Although I was currently unable to find a lawyer to take the case, they didn't know that. I had issues with the medical community after what happened, but I felt it was time I dealt with my inner turmoil by meeting with the people who prompted these feelings. The OB/GYN didn't need to meet with me, and the law was currently on their side, but the fact that they agreed to see me meant a great deal. It wasn't going to be an easy experience for any of us, but it was a meeting that I really needed to ask for and was surprised and relieved they agreed.

As the meeting drew closer, my anxiety escalated. I had continued doing better with sleeping, including the couple days leading up to Denise's death day. However, sleep was sporadic for the night before my meeting with the OB/GYN. I woke up at 4:00 a.m. on the day of the meeting and knew I wouldn't be able to get back to sleep. So I went into the loft and watched part of a movie to relax knowing I would be unable to fall back to sleep.

When it was time to get up, I exercised on the elliptical to reduce my anxiety. It was an emotional morning and my thoughts were all over the place.

I left early to be certain I arrived on time. I dropped off a letter to my personal doctor, letting her know that I was still alive. Her office is in the same vicinity as the OB/GYN's. I was in tears as I walked from my doctor's office to the OB/GYN's.

I checked in and tried to hide my intense emotional state as I sat in the waiting room. After a couple of minutes, I was called and escorted back to the office manager's room where I was greeted by a couple of people.

As I walked into the little office, I met the female doctor who I assumed was the last doctor to see Denise and a gentleman whom I felt I recognized but didn't know. I was originally told it would be the female doctor and the office manager, but I was informed that I would speak with the female doctor and a male doctor. The man was the doctor Denise adored. She always smiled from ear to ear after she saw him, so I always knew immediately which physician had examined her when I picked her up in the parking lot of the prenatal care office building.

I had seen this doctor's face on the number of occasions while I researched and reviewed the various doctors who spent time "caring" for Denise. His had a warm and friendly appearance.

Earlier in the year I had got so tired of being angry with the medical community that I had started writing notes to the people I truly respected. I hated the amount of anger I had with those in the medical profession and finally decided to thank the really good representatives of that community. I had written this man a letter to thank him for treating Denise as the queen she was at the end of her life.

I didn't expect to hear back from him; I felt sure the office had told him not to respond. However, writing to him was something I needed to do. It would be wrong of me to have such hatred for the entire community without identifying the best representatives in it and letting those individuals know how much I cared for how happy they made Denise feel. This doctor was one of the really good ones, and, even if he couldn't reply to me, it was my obligation to thank him for his treatment of Denise.

When he introduced himself, I realized who he was and hugged him and cried on his shoulder. It was clear to the two doctors that I was already an emotional wreck, but I'm sure they were expecting that.

We sat down and they said how very sorry they were for what happened. I imagine it was an excruciating meeting for them, and I tried to make it clear that I wanted to be as honest as I could about what I had been through and all the issues I had with their office as well as the medical community as a whole.

When I was getting ready for the meeting, someone asked me if I had a plan for what I was going to say and what my approach would be. I decided against trying to plan. My main goal was to show them what their decision to not induce Denise had done to me as a man and let them see me for who I was in that moment. I'm sure they quickly got the idea.

I explained to them that my biggest fear was that I would act in a way that made it difficult for them to ever have a meeting with another widower who desperately needed to know what happened as much as I did. I didn't want to be the reason they chose not to help others in a time of grief and anger. I decided to behave in a way that didn't hurt others who might go through the same situation at some point in the future.

They both fully understood. They told me how truly rare it was for them to have to take this type of meeting. Knowing that this was not a common occurrence helped me understand how truly unlikely this was to happen the way that it did. I couldn't imagine anyone else having to go through what I was experiencing and was glad to hear that this was not something that happened often at their office.

I cried in front of these doctors, who probably had a number of other things to do but sat there to comfort me. The male doctor said that when he heard I was going to come in, he had asked to sit in on the meeting with me to better help me cope with my situation. He also mentioned that he had read and kept the letter I wrote to him earlier. I told him how much I appreciated him being there and how much I trusted and respected him for helping me.

I ended up doing most of the talking, but they spoke a fair amount as well. They explained how extremely rare this occurrence was, and I tried to better understand the significance of what *at-risk* means. They let me know that, after looking back through all their information, they determined they would have handled everything the same way. They shared that this highly uncommon accident had affected them deeply.

I told them I had been concerned about the treatment Denise was getting but stayed out of it because I didn't have a medical degree. The male doctor let me know that he was so confident in the other doctors in his office he would feel comfortable bringing his own family members to them, assured they would receive the very best care. I explained my issues with the doctor overseeing Denise's care and shared some of the sad truths I had learned after the fact. There were things I needed to say to them, and afterward there wasn't much anyone could do about our situation.

I could hardly bear being there but was so appreciative of the time they gave me. The male doctor smartly steered the conversation to the human side of things, explaining how desperately he wanted to reach out to me to let me know he had been thinking of me. The hard truth of their situation was they had to be careful about what they said to me. I was able to be completely honest because I wasn't the person that was being looked at for a possible lawsuit. I'm sure there was more they wanted to discuss but were unable to.

It meant so much to me to hear that they struggled personally with what happened and weren't able to let me know they cared. The hard truth was that they didn't show me any support when everything went awful, which left me feeling that the people whom I trusted with the life that was most important to me had let me down. My life was forever tragically altered while they got to go back to their jobs and to their probably wonderful lives. It felt so unjust. They understood where I was coming from, and I recognized where they were coming from.

We also discussed the fact that I had seen Denise immediately following her appointments when she felt she wasn't being heard or respected. She was worried about her pregnancy and expressed her concerns about her health to the office multiple times. I asked why they didn't just deliver those babies when Denise was so worried about her health. They smartly explained that if they delivered every time a mother was concerned, they would have a hospital full of premature babies. I understood this, but their answer felt awkward because I knew I was talking in specifics and they answered with generalization.

I explained that I was talking specifically about a 36-week, at-risk patient whose babies would not have been delivered prematurely. They seemed understanding but couldn't say much more.

The meeting was therapeutic for me. I will always remember how they stuck their necks out to better help me grieve and get over Denise's passing. I didn't agree with everything they said, but I felt so much better knowing they cared and were willing to show compassion to me. They were put in an uncomfortable position but dealt with the issues, both as professionals and as human beings.

I hugged each of the doctors as I left and thanked them for their time. I again mentioned that I hoped I didn't deter them from meeting with someone else in pain like I was. They let me know that I did fine and not to worry about that.

There are really great doctors in the world of medicine, and I told them that each of them was a wonderful representation of that belief. I let them know that if either of them was the doctor who oversaw Denise, and she still would have passed away, my life would be a lot easier because I knew she was given the very best care. Those two doctors represent why people go into medicine, because they have a heart for it. I knew that many of the things I said in that meeting were difficult to swallow given their compassion. However, they accepted my words, and I felt fortunate they agreed to meet with and help me.

As I left, I felt as if a huge weight had been removed from my shoulders. I felt so much better. I knew that some of the people whom I held responsible for Denise's passing cared about me as a person, and that meant the world to me. I was going against a system that had rules which were in place to cover doctors rather than to help people like me. Those doctors and that office set aside some of those rules when they agreed to see me as the grieving person I was rather than as a potential plaintiff in a lawsuit. They might never agree with my statement that it would have been better for their company to see me commit suicide since Denise's death and any potential lawsuit would probably go away if I had. However, after the meeting, I felt much better and I also think that they finally understood my views. Hopefully there would be a better push for making sure that all patients are treated with respect going forward because tomorrow is never guaranteed.

As I drove away, I was so thankful that they cared enough to see me. It was truly amazing how important it was for me to cry in front of them and to know that I mattered to them.

I ran a couple of errands and decompressed before meeting Mrs. Lanane for lunch. She could sense how much better I felt after they showed me the compassion I had needed for so long. I told her all about the meeting, and she was very glad to see how beneficial the experience was for me.

I went ahead and walked around the park after that as I had done the previous year. This time I was by myself, and, although it was lonely, I enjoyed breathing in the fresh air and gazing across the little lake as I strolled over the bridges. It was a really good day.

This would have been our babies' first birthday if things had turned out differently. But our lives had taken a different turn.

I had the chance to talk to a lawyer about the meeting with the doctors. This law firm wasn't going to take the case; they saw me as a man grieving and not a potential plaintiff. It was helpful to hear the legal perspective about the meeting; the attorney seemed to think it was a really great gesture that the OB/GYN's office showed me by meeting. I informed him that I felt much better and would continue to make sure I did my part to keep this kind of tragedy from happening again, but I explained that knowing they cared about my grief brought me some comfort.

I called and picked up Bill and Judy, and we went for ice cream. We each got a single scoop, and like last year I got Denise a scoop of her favorite. Looking at her cup as it sat on the table was sad but something I wanted and needed to do. I have really never cried much while eating ice cream but I did that day.

I told Bill and Judy about the meeting, and they were glad I went and that the OB/GYN office had agreed to sit with me and help me cope with the realities of my life. After we finished our ice cream, I threw away Denise's uneaten treat and we headed home. That night I was joined by my good friend Ryan, the investigator. He once again went out of his way and sat with me while I passed out candy to all the kids and families, who took for granted the life they had.

While the realization that Denise and I would never get to trick-or-treat with our children remained in the corners of my mind, Ryan's presence definitely made the night easier. We sat and talked about sports and movies and laughed a lot. I thanked him and his wife, who ended up passing out candy by herself at their home.

That was a challenging day, but what I experienced also made me feel much more comfortable with life. I definitely slept better that night. I might never agree with everything those doctors said as we sat in their office, but the fact that they took the meeting said a great deal about the people they were. I was glad I didn't confront Denise's main doctor because I don't know how I would have handled it. I was fortunate to sit with two people who were a fantastic representation of what is pure and wonderful about those in the field of medicine.

Chapter 18

Hitting the Wall

After making it through the one-year anniversary of Denise's passing and the kids' first birthday, I had a break approaching. My parents continued to be a really good support system for me. They understood that I needed to have breaks from school and events I could look forward to.

For a while my father had wanted to go to San Francisco, so Mom, Dad, and I had planned a trip for the middle of November to try to take an escape from life. We had a really great time. It is always fun spending time with my parents, and to do so in a city that was as interesting as San Francisco was ideal.

The major highlights of the trip were visiting Alcatraz and getting the opportunity to attend a Golden State Warriors' game. Apart from Mom not feeling great the last day we were there, we had a wonderful time. The vacation was a much-needed break from reality for me. But, as pleasant as trips are, they always come to an end. An empty house and a sad life waited for me upon my return. I dreaded entering that vacant house, but I couldn't deny the sad truth that this was still my life. Of all the times I walked back into the house after a trip, this one was going to be one of the hardest.

There were two different discoveries waiting for me upon my arrival. One was a good surprise and the other was a little disappointing. The first thing that I saw was a letter from someone I wasn't expecting to hear from. One of the two doctors who had met with me at the end of October, sent a letter. Before leaving on the trip, I had written to thank each of them for their time, and she kindly replied to me. I was not expecting this at all and was pretty shocked. I was even more surprised to see that she didn't send it from the office. My first thought was that if her office knew she had sent the letter, they might have reacted unfavorably. Considering that, her gesture meant even more to me. I quickly opened it up and read it to myself. It made me feel really good that she did something that was a human response to a tragedy. Also, this was essentially the first time anyone from that medical office had taken the initiative and reached out to me. To say that receiving and reading that letter was a breath of fresh air would be selling the experience short. I was over the moon that someone who was still employed by a company I held partially responsible for my wife and children's deaths reached out to me. That meant doctors could do the right thing and this doctor was a person who continued to treat people the way she would want to be treated.

She explained how difficult it was meeting with me but said something had changed in her outlook regarding how the medical community had a certain set of rules they must follow because of the current climate of risk management. Through speaking with me, she said she came to realize that this response could make surviving family members' lives much more challenging and even admitted that maybe the medical community needed to rethink how they look at and handle such tragedies. I was floored by how much her words touched me and thankful that my message had changed her outlook. It made me feel good to know that she understood one of the primary reasons I wanted to meet with them.

I honestly don't know if I will ever get a letter that will mean more to me than the one she wrote. I will forever look at her as a continued bright light in the darkness of what I have experienced from the medical community. For the rest of my life, I'll know that letter gave me hope and inspiration that my story could affect people for the better. Even though I still had issues with the OB/GYN whom Denise saw, I could sleep better at night knowing that the last doctor who treated her was a person who cared deeply about her patients and their families. Although the intertwining of our lives was the result of the most terrible of circumstances, I valued her sharing these feelings with me.

As good as I felt about the letter there was something going on inside the house that brought out another emotional response from me. This one, however, prompted the opposite of how I viewed the doctor's letter. After I arrived home, I noticed that a number of furniture pieces had been moved. None of my possessions were taken, so I knew I wasn't the victim of a robbery. But it was obvious that someone had rearranged some of the furniture as well as the mementos I treasured. As I looked around the house, it became clear that Denise's parents had come over while I was gone and cleaned for me. Although this was meant as a kind gesture, many of the furniture pieces were not put back where they were before I left, which was initially alarming.

On the surface this was not a huge deal. But I had a strong desire to keep the house exactly as Denise had left it. Early on, I had been adamant that this continued to be Denise's house. Though more than a year had passed, I had hardly changed anything unless it was absolutely necessary. Other than clearing out the nursery and Denise's clothes, I had really only moved one of the living room chairs. I loved knowing that the house remained just like Denise wanted it.

I had a hard decision about how to handle this situation. On one hand, Denise's parents took time out of their day to clean the house, which was unbelievably nice. On the other hand, I liked how everything was set up and didn't want to alter anything. When I left the house for San Francisco, it was in good shape, and I was happy with my ability to keep it clean.

Denise's parents chose to help in a way that I didn't really want or need. I understood the reason. They were aware of how much time and effort I needed to do all the household chores.

I realized the best way to handle this was to thank them for cleaning the house and leave it there. I decided that if it still bothered me after a few days we would need to work it out as a family.

In my heart I really hoped that I would be able to see the cleaning they did as the kind action they intended it to be. However, as the week went on, I couldn't get past the fact that the house had less Denise in it, which was a tough pill to swallow. At a certain point, I realized that I would need to address the issue and that it was going to be a hard discussion.

To Bill and Judy's credit, they only desired to do something positive for me. If the reason I get upset at someone is because they tried to do something helpful, then that is still a good problem to face. However, this was still an issue I needed to address.

After a couple of days, I texted Bill to ask if they moved anything in the house. He responded that they only repositioned some of the vases they cleaned in the dining room. Even though those vases were moved from where Denise had put them, I didn't spend too much time in that room, so I wasn't really worried about that. What frustrated me was that the living room was changed. Unfortunately, Denise's parents didn't take the responsibility for that, which was the area I hoped they would address.

As I usually try to do, I tried to forget the fact that they weren't truthful with me about an issue that was incredibly dear to my heart. I tried to move on, but again after a couple more days I still felt uneasy about it and decided to speak with them in person.

When I asked if we could have a talk, Bill wondered why. I had no problem letting him know what was bothering me; often I don't like having honest discussions with people who are unaware of the topic, so I was up front about my concerns.

I told him about my frustration with what was done to the house while I was gone, and he agreed to meet with me by himself.

Later that evening, Bill and I spoke and I did much of the talking. I needed him to understand how important this change was to me. I explained that I wanted the furniture to remain as it was when Denise was living and said that it really bothered me when he wasn't honest about what they moved.

He could see the tears in my eyes, and, knowing that it would never get back to the way Denise had decorated it, I'm sure made him feel sad. He acknowledged that he wished they had asked before they cleaned. Bill made a point to say that to clean the house properly, they needed to move some of the furniture, and he was sorry it didn't get moved back to the same exact spot. I told him that I had cleaned around the furniture to avoid this issue. After we discussed the current situation, I brought up something else I didn't want to talk about but I knew I needed to.

By this point Denise and the babies had been gone for about 13 months. Bill and Judy were probably two of the most dedicated people in respect to staying with me through all of this time. One of the sad truths about where I was in my grieving was I was really struggling with the limited amount I heard from people. Friends asked me how the one-year anniversary went, and I replied that it was good to hear from so many people who cared but added that it really hurt when I heard from nobody two days later. People had gotten back to their lives, and I didn't do a very good job of letting them know I was still in pain. I had isolated myself in hopes that others could live happy lives without dwelling on my daily struggles and desperate loneliness. It hurt even more when I didn't hear from people.

Bill and Judy were by far the people who best understood all of this, and, when we had this issue, it made me realize I couldn't continue to go on with the current life I was living. I had "hit a wall," and I knew I needed to do a much better job of taking care of myself and spend less time trying to make sure other people were happy.

Bill and Judy shouldn't have been the tipping point for my emotions, but they were because they were the ones I felt safe with, and they were the people who continued to be with me through this horrible journey. It was a really hard spot for me but one I knew I needed to step back from and properly address.

I informed Bill that I needed to take a break from them and really gather myself together. I hated the fact that this was the week before Thanksgiving and a couple of days later was Judy's 70th birthday that I would miss. However, I recognized that I had to address these growing concerns that I was having regarding my current support system. I also needed to take a break from Bill and Judy so they could truly appreciate how real my frustrations were and that this wasn't something I would get over quickly.

I'm sure it was hard for Bill to hear this, but I had to take this step. I still loved Bill and Judy; they will always have a special place in my heart. However, in order to ensure we shared a better relationship in the future, I had to make the short-term decision to back away from them for the time being. I will always regret that I wasn't around for that holiday and birthday because I knew we should have been together as the family we tried to be.

On Thanksgiving, the gym wasn't open, so I went for a lovely walk and then to visit Denise's niche. I spoke to her as I always did and apologized for not being with her family for the holiday. I also said that I hoped she would understand my reasons and see it from my side. It was a difficult decision, but I knew I needed to take better steps to help my healing; this was one of the unhappy truths of the uphill climb I continued to make.

I spent Thanksgiving dinner with my neighbors, Tricia and Adam. I ate more food than I normally do, but I felt at ease and comforted by their family, who had already done so much for me. I couldn't think of anyone else I would rather have been with other than Denise's family.

Breaks from my students were always challenging, but I kept myself as busy as I could with a number of projects. I made a photobook of our trip to San Francisco that I hoped to include with my parents Christmas presents. I also continued working on a Lego project that would serve as a Christmas present for the same wonderful family who hosted me for Thanksgiving.

I continued to spend the last moments of each night working on my writings to Denise. I had spent so many hours writing to her or about our story that I didn't know what else to do. My most recent efforts involved reading over and editing the daily journal I did during the six months after she passed. I reached the last entry and edited the final letter and didn't know what to do after that.

I still found myself incapable of walking away from the practice of ending my day sharing my heart with Denise.

During the Thanksgiving holiday, I decided that I would re-edit my nightly reflections because I didn't know what else to do. Even though I had just looked over them recently, the thought of moving farther away from Denise was something I still wasn't ready to do.

With Thanksgiving concluded, I knew it was time to start taking matters related to my grieving into my own hands. There were conversations I needed to have with many of the family and friends Denise and I were close to.

My first phone call was to one of Denise's best friends, Amy's husband, Russ. Amy spoke at Denise's funeral and Russ was a pallbearer. I hadn't spoken to Russ for a while or heard much from him in the longest time. As I was re-reading my journal, I saw a line I had written about how he did such a great job in setting up our memorial fund. I wanted to first make sure he knew how much I appreciated him setting up the fund before I broached the difficult discussion of his recent lack of connection.

I texted him and asked if there would be a time soon when we could catch up. He quickly let me know that he would be around that weekend, and the next day we were able to talk.

I was worried about how to approach these difficult issues because it wasn't like I was mad at him and didn't want to come across that way. But I was hurt that I hadn't heard from him much. I understood I had a significant role in this since I had not done a good job of reaching out to others myself. This conversation was not about his lack of support but about how neither of us had communicated how we were doing during those many months. I just hoped I could articulate it without offending him.

Denise had lived with Amy and Russ for some time before she met me, and he was always one of the friendliest and most personable people I ever met. Once I was able to get him on the phone, I first thanked him for what he did for our memorial fund, and he assured me I had already thanked him enough but he continued to be glad of the fact I appreciated what he had done. Then I carefully mentioned that I hadn't heard from him in a while and said it was hard on me. I was curious as to how he would handle his response because our conversation could go either of two ways.

To Russ' amazing credit, we were able to have an open conversation about how we were both doing. He even articulated that he didn't really know what to say to me, so he just tried not to bother me. It was a reflective and heartfelt conversation. We were both sympathetic to the other person's point of view and aware of each of our own faults related to the current situation. Russ was incredibly sincere, which put my mind at ease. Because of how well he handled himself, I was able to open up to him and to talk to him about what I was going through. I remain so grateful to Russ and hope he understood how much our honest and deeply tough conversation not only relieved me but also helped me know how to approach the difficult exchanges with other friends that lay ahead.

After my honest discussion with Russ, I was able to speak with Denise's other good friend Kelly's husband, Gus. Kelly too spoke at Denise's funeral and Gus was a pallbearer. But the two of them lived within 10 minutes of me whereas Amy and Russ resided across the country. Several months earlier Kelly and Gus each had visited and sat with me at the empty house for a lengthy span, but at a certain point I didn't hear much from them.

I was frank with Gus about the fact that I still needed to hear from him and also acknowledged that many of the issues I was experiencing resulted from my own mishandling of my grief. I needed to be less fake around others. How I had appeared in public gave friends the impression I was doing okay when in truth my healing was still progressing, and getting over the loss of Denise and the kids was something I continued to deal with every day and would for a long time to come. He was understanding and again I was proud that Denise and I had such good people in our lives who were willing to engage in an honest and difficult discussion.

Later that week I spoke with Denise's sister and brother-in-law, Dawn and Brian, and they too handled themselves remarkably well. I did not want to sound as if I were accusing others of moving on and forgetting about me. I just needed to hear from them. Dawn and Brian both related to my situation. As tough as their lives were, they realized that being able to come home to each other and interact with their daughter Sara helped tremendously. Since I didn't have that, they knew it was much more difficult for me. They too were insightful and again I was grateful that no one thought I was blaming others for not reaching out. They recognized that I was at a point in my healing journey when I needed to have honest conversations with those closest to me so I could continue to progress.

By making the rounds, talking to people, and opening myself up, I was hoping that I could handle myself better than I had done with Bill and Judy. I was still disappointed about that. I had too many negative emotions inside me, and, when our issue arrived, it was more a reflection of my feelings getting the better of me. They were trying to do something thoughtful, and, although I appreciated it, I made a bigger deal over the issue because I had allowed myself to become so isolated and guarded with those who were close to Denise and me. It was only a matter of time before my volcano erupted. I was just glad I avoided the kind of inappropriate emotional outburst I had the previous Christmas. I knew it was time to stop withdrawing from others as I had done so many times before.

Although Bill, Judy, and I were going through a rough patch in our relationship, I felt we would be okay in the long run because of how we handled an uncomfortable situation. While I missed Thanksgiving and Judy's 70th birthday, we were entering the Christmas season, and we all needed to be together then because, as wonderful as Christmas is for most people, for us it was challenging. Like last year, this holiday was going to be painful.

Chapter 19

Christmas

The holiday season has always been one of the favorite times of the year for almost everyone. But at this point in my journey, "everyone" did not include me. The December after Denise passed was utterly miserable, and I wasn't sure how this year was going to be. I anticipated a month of sorrow but believed my emotional state likely would be less intense than during the previous year's darkness.

It took some time but Bill, Judy, and I became friendlier. After a couple of weeks of us sitting together in church we started to feel more comfortable with each other again. Bill and Judy were always welcoming on Sundays when we were close to each other. It took a little while for me to open up to them. I normally don't say much to many people in church, including Bill and Judy. However, once my anger cleared and I realized that a large part of the reason I was still here was because they never forgot about my daily struggle, I was able to move past our conflict.

One day as we were leaving church, I asked them if it would be okay if I stopped over for dinner. They seemed delighted and let me know that they would enjoy my company. That evening we had a normal dinner and got back to our former selves.

It felt right to be back together with Bill and Judy. As frustrated as I had been, I knew we needed to face the upcoming challenge of getting through the holidays as a family.

When Bill, Judy, and I had discussed how we would handle things this year, I said that I could really do without the holidays, but unfortunately Christmas was going to happen in any case. Again this year we attended the church service for people who are going through grief or hard times. I remembered going through a number of tissues to dry my tears the previous Christmas. This year I felt slightly less depressed and lonely, but I still had to hold my emotions a few times during the service to keep them from getting the better of me.

The day after the service for the bereaved was my last day with students before the break. I recalled crying in my car the previous year as everyone else left for the holidays to be with their families. I was pleasantly surprised that I didn't cry at the end of the day this time. I just collected all my belongings and set out what I wanted to work on the next day during my workday before driving to go to my weekly therapy appointment.

The following day I worked for about three hours before I went to lunch and a movie with my assistant principal. We had planned to hang out for a while since we both had some work that day. It was a good little escape and something that I looked forward to. I realized that I wasn't getting nearly as emotional as I had the year before, and part of me felt uncomfortable with that fact.

I was making progress and glad to be moving forward in my grief. Yet, a large part of me still believed I should be at home in the fetal position so overcome with grief that I couldn't function. I knew that Denise would want me to get out and be around people, but I still felt odd that I was functioning without her. I knew I would continue to deal with this feeling going forward. Her passing still felt so wrong as did moving on without her.

After the movie, I came home to spend about ten days without seeing my students and without the structure school provided. I continued to be blessed that my job provided so much support for me, but I also knew that having these breaks could be challenging. Removing that stable outlet provided a test to see how far I had actually come.

During the first holiday season without Denise, I didn't put up any decorations. Apart from a couple of unwrapped presents for Denise, nothing inside or outside the house gave the impression that Christmas was coming. Even though I still wasn't in the holiday spirit a year later, I needed to take steps toward the progress I knew I was capable of making. I still couldn't bring myself to put up Denise's Christmas tree, and, God help me, I was still nowhere near the point where I could have opened the attic and looked through all her ornaments. Instead I went to Target and purchased an $8 small white Christmas tree. I didn't want to spend too much money, knowing that whatever I bought would be put into the trash the day after Christmas.

By the small tree I had a few presents that I bought for myself. Most were just articles of clothing that I needed. I got myself some new athletic socks, dress socks, and black athletic shorts. I also purchased a couple of new disc golf Frisbees in hopes of using those to get out of the house every once in a while.

My parents wrapped some presents for me as well, and I put them under the little tree. I ended up buying Denise a DVD and a calendar that had pictures of cute animals that I knew she would have loved. I didn't put up any stockings or any other decorations. Only a few other presents for family members and friends lay under the tree.

I still was far from being in the holiday spirit, but I recognized the value of making steps forward with respect to probably the hardest holiday for someone living with the type of sadness I had.

Now that I was a lot more comfortable around Denise's family, we all agreed to do our annual gift exchange at Bill and Judy's house on Christmas Eve. It was good being with Bill, Judy, Dawn, Brian, and Sara. Whenever we were together, we usually had a wonderful time. We carried on our tradition of the grown-ups exchanging presents, and, apart from Bill getting replicas of about three of his gifts, everything went well. We enjoyed eating lasagna and then got ready to go to church for the Christmas Eve service.

As usual, we arrived in plenty of time. I put my water down and went to the bathroom before heading out to Denise's niche. This evening, I really had a hard time and cried a lot. The sound of brass instruments playing in the background to welcome churchgoers made it difficult to compose my thoughts. I found it frustrating because I greatly wanted to talk to Denise. The musicians were excellent but extremely loud. I couldn't seem to concentrate as much as I would have liked and think it made the evening more difficult for me.

I sat there shivering from the winter chill despite being bundled up. Hearing the jubilant music and people who happily walked by only added to the sense of coldness. I went into the church earlier than I normally would to visit the restroom and clear the tears from my face.

By this point, I cared little about whether people could see I had been crying. If they noticed, then they saw the real me. Nonetheless, because it was supposed to be a joyous occasion, I felt obligated, at least on Christmas Eve, to give them their happy day.

As expected, the church service proved difficult. Again I tried to hold my head high and keep my emotions somewhat in check. One of the challenges during this time of the year was listening to the often-repeated "Joy to the World." Although it's a beautiful song, after hearing it that first Christmas alone, I easily could have happily never heard that song again.

This year the song was sung a number of times in the lead-up to the holiday and during that service. It was awful, but it wasn't as heartbreaking as it was the previous year. I still hated the song, but I was at a better place to try and sit through it.

After the service, I went back out to the niche and sat there a little bit more. I told Denise I would see her in the morning and headed home. I knew that the next day would be depressing, but I kept reminding myself that it probably wouldn't be as bad as last year. I would be making the rounds to some really hard places and hoped I would get enough sleep to help me withstand the experience.

The next morning I woke fairly early, took a shower, and put a couple of my Christmas presents away.

My first destination was Denise's niche. I quickly stopped by to tell her and the babies merry Christmas. The columbarium was the only place I wanted to be at that moment in this cruel world. But I had other errands, so I only stayed about five minutes before heading to Dawn and Brian's to watch Sara open her presents.

Upon arriving there, I put my gifts by her other ones and tried to interact with the family. Earlier in the month, I had reached out to Dawn about a couple book ideas for Sara. All along I knew I wanted to buy presents for Sara that Denise would have given her. Since Denise was a teacher, many of the gifts she bought Sara were engaging and educational. I had gotten Sara a little watch since she seemed to like the one I wore, a couple of chapter books, Lego sets, and something else Sara asked for: educational workbooks.

Surprisingly, she seemed to enjoy all of my presents. Even though they weren't the most expensive ones she received, she appeared to appreciate them, which made me feel good.

As I sat down watching Sara open her gifts, I checked my phone occasionally. I had gotten a couple of texts from friends. Most of the messages said, "Merry Christmas." I really don't know what to tell people who say those words to me. This was not going to be a "merry" holiday.

This was another example of the fine line I needed to walk. On one hand, I wanted to appreciate that people were reaching out and acknowledging me. On the other hand, I didn't want to give others the impression that I was doing fine and end up further isolating myself as a result. I chose my words carefully to remind people of the truth of my situation. Some people replied; others did not. One wonderful person just acknowledged the sadness of that day. This made me feel understood. Even so, I had no desire to take happiness from others, so I had to walk the tight rope between letting them know my truth and not bringing them into my sorrow. I still wasn't in a place for happiness even on this "joyous" occasion.

As Sara continued opening her presents, I had a little food but avoided drinking many liquids since I would be making a couple of stops before I got home. I just hoped that, with the range of emotions I faced, I wouldn't get a headache.

Once Sara finished opening her presents, and before Dawn and Brian started unwrapping theirs, I quickly gave them hugs and said my goodbyes.

I returned to Denise's niche to spend more time than I had earlier. As I sat there talking to Denise, I told her about Sara's presents and how much she seemed to enjoy them. I shared that I tried to purchase gifts I thought she herself would have bought, carrying on her legacy to honor Denise's beautiful heart and kind intentions even in the little things. Sitting there in the cold, sad, and alone, I didn't have anywhere else I wanted or needed to be.

I showed Denise the Christmas presents I got for her and then read the two cards I picked out for her. It was hard finding cards that could say what I wanted to share with her since our situation was unique, but I usually found something along the lines of what I felt was appropriate. I read her the notes that I wrote inside each one. It was intensely difficult, but I was determined to make it through.

While I sat there, my mind wandered to what our kids would have wanted this year for Christmas. As much as I missed Denise, she wasn't the only life that was lost. I never knew what to say as I sat there beside their ashes. I just spoke from the heart. I told Denise how much I loved her and the babies and wished them merry Christmas again before I returned to the car.

My next stop was to Denise's school. I parked at the back of her school and went over to her bench. I was crying quite a bit along the way. That beautifully-crafted bench was a wonderful way to honor Denise. I sat there feeling despondent. Although I had already spoken to Denise at the niche, coming to her bench brought me an added sense of closeness to the woman she was, the woman I will always love. After remaining there looking out over the parking lot, I got myself together and strode back to the car to drive home.

At that time of the day, there weren't many cars on the road. Most everyone had already reached their destination and were with their families. I was on my way back to an empty house that was built for four in my car that was bought for four.

After I arrived, I changed my clothes, grabbed the case that held Denise's video, and put it in the DVD player. I sat on the couch in silence watching the parade of snapshots of a life filled with love and happiness. This wonderful film was a testament to a woman I hadn't seen in over a year but who still lived in my heart. As the photo of her during her first trimester approached, I felt my emotions intensify as they always did. I hadn't seen the film in over two months, but I knew the order of pictures by memory after so many viewings. When that picture came onto the screen, I howled as I always do and tried to bring myself together as quickly as I could so that I didn't miss any of her beautiful smiles.

Denise was so full of life. As long as I'd known her, she was really happy. All she ever wanted was to be a mother, and she would have been an incredible one. All of those photos demonstrated how wonderful she was with kids and in general. As the film ended, once again I acknowledged how much better I was doing than I had during the previous year, a fact that both gratified and saddened me. I wanted to progress but I didn't want to think it was ever okay that I wouldn't see Denise again in this life. Every bit of forward movement brought its own emotional battle, and I remained heartbroken.

After I put the DVD away, I grabbed all our photo albums and sat on the couch, looking through them in chronological order. Seeing all our trips and little activities we shared made me smile. Some of these pictures made it into the film but a majority did not. I turned the pages of our wedding album and viewed so many family members whom I had not seen since the week after Denise passed.

I sat with a warm cup of tea and took my time looking at the images of our past. Seeing those snapshots made me happy, not because I was managing but because I knew we had lived a wonderful five years. I was so thankful that we documented our lives with so many photos, keepsakes to always remember. I imagined flipping through the pages of these albums with Denise as we showed our kids our life before they appeared. Denise and I took on projects that reflected the very best of who we were together, and I was proud that we had so many of these moments recorded to always remind me of the love she and I shared.

Once I got through all the pictures, I went ahead and put the photobooks away and started working on the tasks I wanted to complete over my break. With the long break from work, I never planned to just sit and relax, so I started a list of all the jobs I wanted to complete. I ended up with over 40 jobs, some which would take multiple hours and others about ten minutes. I went ahead and worked on some of these until Dad arrived.

During previous discussions with my parents about how we would treat Christmas, I had explained that I needed to stay in town because there was some work here I wanted to complete. They originally wanted me to visit them but understood my desire to remain at home. Mom had planned on coming to see me, but she wasn't going to be able to make it because she was scheduled to play piano during the holiday church services.

About a week before Christmas, Dad informed me that he would like to come. I realized that if I continued to fill the hard times with people, I really wouldn't be able to fully understand what my life would be like without Denise. But I couldn't bring myself to tell Dad not to come for a few days. I couldn't deny him his duty of being a loving father and told him I would be more than happy to see him.

Dad understood that I would be working on numerous projects and that his trip wouldn't be as enjoyable as it could be. He assured me that he would be bringing his own work to keep him busy.

It was really great to see Dad again. We hadn't been together since September when I went to San Francisco with my parents. Dad and I spent the evening catching up and talking about how we each were doing. Very quickly I remembered what a joy it was to just have someone at the house to share meals and conversation.

Dad did a wonderful job of both respecting my need to complete tasks and finding ways we could spend time together. We agreed to go to a movie one day, and Dad even accompanied me to my weekly therapist visit. I got a great deal of my work done while Dad was there and he helped me begin one of my next projects.

I had told Dad that I had planned on throwing away many of the Lego architecture sets that I built the previous year, but, after hearing from a couple of people, I decided to take them apart so I could give them to others who might enjoy assembling them. I wisely kept all of the instructions. Dad said he would be more than happy to get started on that project, and, during his time at the house, he disassembled about five of the sets.

I would take apart the remainder of them after he left, giving me another project to keep me busy. Between work and planning the 5K race again for the following year, I had plenty to do. Breaking down the Legos proved meaningful to me. I would be destroying something that represented the worst time in my life when I struggled with Denise's death. I hoped that someone else could get some enjoyment out of assembling them. For me, I was removing another reminder of a period I wished I could forget.

The day before New Year's Eve, I was asked by one of my good friends if I would be interested in going to a Duke basketball game. Always a sports fan, I was excited about attending the game. Dad had left that morning and, although it was tough seeing him go, I was relieved that I didn't shed too many tears. Anticipation of going to the Duke game drew my focus away from my sadness for a while.

One of my goals was to be more social during the coming year and try to find some happiness in this world. Denise wouldn't want me to be sad for the rest of my life, but I still didn't know how to balance the desire to experience joy with the big picture of my still depressing life.

Going to the Duke game and having a really great time helped me to realize that, going into the next year, I needed to embrace and try to live in the happy moments. I was always uncomfortable when I tried to accomplish this during the past year. Trying to be happy was something I had to work at going forward. Somehow I had to find a way to live a second life, one without the woman I loved.

Having a blast at that basketball game brought me hope. My friend was so gracious to get me out of the house and remind me that I used to have fun. As I sought to find ways to move on with my life, I knew I had to cultivate this ability to simply enjoy those moments and focus only on the short term, on the present moment. I had to try not to worry about the long term.

At the end of the game, I returned home to the empty house and, yes, it was still lonely and sad, but at least I appreciated and got the most out of that game and the joy it gave to me.

I also learned something else when I got home. Because I arrived later than I normally do, I had my dinner later. As a result of my breaks in structure, I hadn't slept my normal hours that week. That night as expected I had to get up a couple of times to go to the restroom and couldn't get back to sleep. I had been making improvements, but I still desperately required the structure to continue to perform at the levels I had become accustomed to. I wasn't at a place yet where I could pull away the ordered system I had put in place.

The next day was New Year's Eve and I continued working on my list of tasks. I didn't feel like celebrating. My resolution for the year before was to survive and I did that. My reward was continuing to live this sad life and heal enough so that, if an opportunity ever presented itself to find the kind of love I had with Denise, I would be ready for it.

Although I was definitely better than the previous year, I still had little to celebrate. I went to bed early because I needed to function. I had made it through the year, and, although there were some really bad times, I could look back on them knowing I was taking the necessary steps to move forward even if that meant being forced to continue to get farther away from Denise.

Chapter 20

Looking Back and Looking Forward

With the New Year presenting itself, so did the realization that I was going to have to live a new life. Denise and I were incredibly happy and what happened to us will stick with me for the rest of my life. In a million years, I never would have thought that this tragedy would have occurred. Even though I know how cliché it sounds, it still seems like a horrible nightmare.

I hated the idea of moving on but knew I had to keep making those steps forward. I kept my resolution the previous year: to remain alive. This year I would attempt to be more social. It was important for me to deconstruct the extreme structure I had built in order to make it through; part of that meant placing myself into more social situations. I still had no idea what to say to people when questions arose about what happened to Denise. There was no good answer to how a pregnant woman at full-term passed away. I would need to prepare for these kinds of inquiries even if I still had no way to answer them.

I had built this cocoon to isolate myself so that I could get back to a place where I could function and manage my emotions. With the new year, I had to move forward even if that meant facing the pain of leaving Denise in the past. This concept weighed heavily on me. Being in this position when I still had so many pieces of the heart to mend seemed impossible.

The first step forward came on the evening of New Year's Day. I had continued ending all of my days with something related to Denise. I had spent so many nights writing to her and typing our story. Because I wasn't ready to move away from her, I re-edited many of the writings. As I worked through my nightly reflections, I started counting the days remaining in December. It seemed fitting that the last day of my editing would be New Year's Eve. I didn't plan for it but knew that it was the way it was supposed to be.

As I reviewed my journaling to Denise that night, I felt odd that I was going to be removing another support system that kept her memory alive. Removing that nightly ritual was a step forward I needed to take.

New Year's Day was not as bad as I thought it would be. An evening of watching college football offered a welcome distraction. It felt wrong to use the game as a means of escape. I believed I needed to pull away from the kinds of distractions that had helped me survive in the worst pit of despair I had ever known.

That night I didn't get up out of bed and go to the computer. Instead I just turned the television off and reached for my book. The football game went longer than expected, and I was able to fall asleep after my routine of reading for a half hour.

The next evening it felt odd not going back into the den to complete my evening routines. But I understood it was part of the process of letting go of my supports. Even so, it continued to feel *wrong*.

As my coping systems fell away, I reflected on a number of things. I thought a great deal about how this tragedy happened and looked at how I found my place in this horrible life.

Instead of being there when Denise needed me most, I leaned on those who we are supposed to trust and allowed them to take control of my wife's health. Because we had been through so much to get to that place, I felt confident that everything would end up the way it should. When it all went wrong, I was completely pathetic and unprepared for the challenges.

I believed in those doctors even though they didn't treat Denise with the respect she deserved. I believed God would see us through what should have been the happiest time of our lives. I always assumed that the conflict with the doctor's office would be something that we joked about years later. However, it didn't turn out like that. I used to pray daily for healthy babies, and, when everything played out, I realized I was praying for the wrong thing.

God and I still have our issues. I may never view God the way others do. I know I will always wonder why He didn't prevent this when I believe He had the power to. I no longer have the anger that drew me to want to punch God in the face. However, I know that when I die the first thing I will do is to hug Denise and those kids. I will then say hello to all those people who had fallen before me. After that, I will be going to God and asking Him the same question I have asked since Denise died, "Why didn't you prevent this?" That question still plagues me as it has since she left this world.

If I seem more religious than I was before Denise's passing, it's because I want to believe that Denise is happy up in heaven. Denise deserved the best. She deserved to be a mother to those children here on Earth. Since that was taken from her, I just hope that she is up in heaven with those kids looking down on me, happy that I'm managing to survive in this world.

Although I still struggle with my views on God and religion, I will continue to go to church because that is where Denise is. I don't cry as much as I once did but I still feel incredibly sad. I know that when I die, whether that's relatively soon or many years from now, my ashes will be placed next to those of Denise and our babies. I will always feel that God had a part in this tragedy and may never know how much. I still feel that he had the power to prevent it and that sadly he didn't intervene.

I have the most frustration with the doctors and the medical community who took our money and failed to give her the best care possible. When Denise died, I was so dumbfounded. I had no idea what to say or how to act. I desperately needed to hear from those doctors and to know they cared for her and then for me. I never got that. I do believe this was a freak accident, but I also think those doctors followed a flawed system built on knowing the data and specific structures for evaluating patients. When it came down to it, the data is what killed her.

The data said she was okay and that was good enough for the doctors.

Denise expressed her concerns to two different doctors the week before she died, and both sent her away. The last visit she had was probably the hardest moment for me to understand. Trying to calm Denise in the parking lot enough to go upstairs to the prenatal appointment was really hard. I should have handled that exchange differently, marched right back to the OB/GYN and done whatever I could. But I trusted the medical professionals, and in the end they sat idle without offering me any type of support while I tried to deal with their mistake.

I never wanted money and I still don't. To me it would be blood money. I only ever really cared about making sure this didn't happen to anyone else. If they say sorry and only I know about it, that doesn't change things as much as a lawsuit that put Denise's death in the news could. Doctors are meant to help people. But Denise's voice and concerns over her and the babies' well-being didn't even matter. She told me her concerns and she communicated them to those doctors. When her medical records were given to me and there was not even the mention of her concern even though I knew she expressed them to multiple doctors, I was appalled at the injustice.

When I tried to put myself in the shoes of those in that doctor's office, I found it really hard. Had I been one of them, I would have demanded to reach out. Instead, during the worst time in my life, the people I trusted with Denise's health, who may or may not have treated her the way she deserved, went into risk management. They showed me they cared more about their business and money than for my wellbeing.

I still believe that it would have been better for them if I had committed suicide. They clearly were instructed to not contact me for fear of saying something that would put them into legal jeopardy. If I had died, that issue would have evaporated.

As much anger as I still have toward the medical community, I find myself in a unique situation. I'm sure people will always view me as someone who hates the medical profession. I don't see it like that. I believe this story could be used to help others. I had asked to speak at a couple of medical conferences, and, although my emails were ignored, I doubt there are too many other people who can speak to the need for patient and family care as well as I can.

I hate the fact that Denise is gone. She and I both believed in education and in trying to make the world a better place. I may never get the opportunity to share my story and do my part to instill the need to listen to patients and give them the respect they need and deserve. However, I suspect the part of this tragedy that troubles people is that this story represents the biggest fear to the medical profession. Denise's story demonstrates that doctors have really hard jobs. They follow the tests and the systems that have been put in place. Those systems help *almost* everyone. Denise was the exception.

I have spoken to various individuals since Denise's passing about this. Some people whom I greatly trust have told me that this was probably a freak accident but that those doctors gave her proper care. Hearing this fills me with a range of emotions. My feelings are clouded by the fact that *she* didn't feel great about the care she received, and clearly her concerns over her body didn't warrant any type of medical documentation. But it also makes me hopeful that this doesn't happen often and was truly a rare occurrence. I hope and pray that no one ever goes through losing his or her whole life the way I did.

Looking back on everything, Denise may have been given *adequate* care. But passable care wasn't what she needed.

While I was meeting with someone about the estate paperwork, a wonderful lady mentioned to me something that I have pondered a great deal since. She revealed that when she was pregnant with her child, she was asked to wear a heart rate monitor. I have thought back many times about this, wondering if a heart rate monitor was something that could have helped Denise.

I believe it likely would have. I'm not saying that the monitor would have saved her life, but I can say with almost total certainty that she would have gladly worn one. It would have been at least some additional support and would have provided data to indicate what was happening before and at the time of her death. If Denise still had died with a heart rate monitor, at least I would have slept better knowing something was in place to check on her health between doctor's visits. This small precaution would have been far better than just sending her out the door and hoping she made it back the next week. Again, I'm looking at all of this through the lens of hindsight, the only way I can at this point. Denise would have wanted me to learn from this sad experience and help others avoid a similar fate.

With everything that I feel toward the medical profession, I fully recognize the challenges they face daily. I imagine few careers have higher risks or higher rewards. I had seen an ugly side of the medical community that few encounter. This gives me a unique perspective that affects how I perceive others in the medical field and probably will for the rest of my life. It is my responsibility to make sure I thank those who conduct themselves the *right* way instead of taking them for granted. I believe people should be treated the way they would want to be. However, common courtesy doesn't always come the way I expect it to. I will do my best to make sure I let those who do their jobs the right way receive the proper thanks. We need great people making the decisions that affect all of us. We also need to be treated with the respect and care we deserve. When that doesn't happen, it makes tragedies like this so much harder to live with.

I know I would have slept better had I known Denise was given the best care possible from each of her doctors. Unfortunately, sleep was scarce and my life was harder knowing Denise felt she wasn't heard by her physicians.

There are wonderful and outstanding people in the medical profession, and I have seen a number of these people. But because of my experience, I know I have an obligation to make sure they continue to give everyone the best of care.

Many of the best doctors, nurses, technicians, etc. listen to their patients and treat people with the respect they themselves would want. Maybe my voice can remind people how fragile life is and that we need to encourage those who give their best effort in the medical field and in every profession.

I will continue to express gratitude to doctors and nurses who seem to really care about their patients. I may have seen the worst side of the medical community, but I won't allow myself to *only* see the worst.

As I continued to look back on all that transpired after Denise's passing, I recognized a few things that really helped me survive. Some of these were internal factors and others were external. These beliefs and tools that helped me to endure deserve to be given voice, so it is only right to mention them and why they helped me.

Teaching kids and working for the school where I taught was the single greatest factor in my ability to continue to live. My students brought me so much joy, and my responsibility to them gave me an outlet for success. For the longest while, I thought the students didn't view me as a guy grieving. However, as time went on, I realized that it was my view that changed when I was with them. In their presence, I didn't see myself as a grieving person. My kids were the single best thing in my life and my love of teaching those students will always be the biggest factor in my survival.

The next external aid came from podcasts. Leaving work each day and coming home to a house that was completely empty was terrible. But I was supported by the many podcasts I listened to. They greatly helped me keep my head up and be engaged. As I listened to them, I felt less alone. Often the most painful times for me happened in the shower because I couldn't hide from my life in there. Podcasts seemed to distract me from a world that I didn't belong in. So thank you, Bill Simmons, Malcolm Gladwell, and the many contributors to the Ringer podcasts who filled hours upon hours of alone time and helped me feel less empty and lonely.

Mr. Bob will always go down as one of the single biggest reasons I made it out alive. Mr. Bob was brought into my world by the church. Having someone with whom I could be open about all my anger and sadness was highly therapeutic. From the beginning, I recognized the value of releasing the emotions that tended to build up inside me. My weekly walks with Mr. Bob gave me the outlet I needed. Because he didn't know Denise, he provided a different perspective that I desperately needed. He understood that there were times I didn't want to talk about Denise. We found a common interest in North Carolina State athletics and movies that could fill our time together, allowing me to talk even when there wasn't anything I wanted to say about my current situation. Bob was a blessing and one I will always credit to the church.

The last external factor that had a great impact on my survival was the structure I created around me and the time I spent at the gym. I desperately needed to find some type of routine to provide focus. I tried so desperately to keep myself going and this organized, rigid approach to life anchored me in the task at hand and in the moment. Working out at the gym or on the elliptical at home enabled me to release anger and anxiety and rid my body of pent-up emotions. Taking care of my body in this way was a necessary step toward healing emotionally.

My internal beliefs helped me get to a point where I could see the world much differently than I did after the tragedy occurred. The first conviction was that this tragedy had taken three lives and it was on me to make sure it didn't take four. I felt strongly that Denise would have been upset if I would have joined her soon after she left this world. I understood this tragedy shouldn't have happened but it did, and, if I went down a bad road, then I would have no one to blame but myself. It was true that I was put in an incredibly difficult situation, but it was my responsibility to figure out how to make the best of it and move on with my life.

The second idea that kept me going was the understanding that if I passed away the voice of Denise would be silenced. While I realized her family would have stepped in and done a great job, Denise was my wife. We spent five unbelievable years together, and I felt it was my moral obligation to carry on her legacy and to help this world remember one of its rising stars.

Denise was such a wonderful person and what happened to her will always be wrong. But I wanted people to remember her for the bright light that she was in this world, for how she lived and not how she died.

Finally, I felt that there was a fight that needed to happen, an injustice that had to be addressed so that others would never have to face this kind of experience. Although this didn't come to fruition, the belief that the world had to learn something from this tragedy helped me carry on past the incredible sorrow that overwhelmed my being during the year after her passing. Early on when everything was so bad, I truly believed something could be done. That belief kept me moving forward. Although it didn't play out the way I wished, it still helped me continue to crawl out of the darkness and kept me surviving.

Denise and I had something that was truly wonderful. I hated the way things turned out, the ending to the life we worked so hard to build. The loss of my wife and unborn twins continues to haunt me. Still, if someone had told me the ending and that I would only have a five-year journey with Denise, I would have chosen to follow that path in a heartbeat. Denise and I had something that was special. We had true love. We almost had everything any family could want—until it all went so wrong. Yes, I hated how it all ended, but, knowing what I know now, I still would have gone on the ride with Denise even though we didn't get to experience our highest of highs and even though I alone had to face the lowest of lows.

Since I have done a thorough job of looking back, it's only fitting that I attempt to gaze ahead. Of course, this is much, much harder. I have no idea what my future holds. I only know I will attempt to show up every day to teach the kids who brought me so much joy even during the worst time of my life. Although I can experience happiness at school and be grateful for my ability to teach those kids, my sadness is far from over. I will have to face more challenging issues soon and still don't know if I'm fully ready for the next stage of my life.

Denise's life and death will be with me always. I will forever wonder about the life she and I lost. I hate the fact that Denise never got to hold those children and read to them here in the physical world. This universe did a wrong when it took away Denise and those kids. This tragedy will follow me until the day I die. Each day I am reminded what others have and take for granted—and what I lost. I will always see families together and know that I would give anything to have that with Denise.

These issues will linger years to come, if not for the rest of my life. I understand the need to continue letting out this pain and will continue to go to therapy for a long time. Since the day of this greatest loss, I've valued the ability to talk to someone and that belief likely won't change.

A number of hurdles lie ahead, and with all of the others I will have to face and attempt to overcome them. The main one will be having to live a second life since my first life with Denise, the only one I wanted, was taken from me. I have no idea if I can build a new life or how I will handle the moving on beyond Denise. I simply know Denise would want me to be happy, so for her I will try.

I decided to keep the car we purchased with the thought of bringing our babies home from the hospital. But I have no idea what will happen to the house. It represents the life she and I strived to build and reminds me of all that was taken from us. I continue to sleep in our bed. Sadly, I still need to continue to keep an air freshener in the room so I am not reminded of the worst moment of my life.

For now, Denise's degrees that she worked so hard for and photographs of our joyful moments still hang on the wall. At some point I'm sure that they will all be taken down, but I don't look forward to those sad moments. Bill built a chest to hold the keepsakes of our beautiful life; I worry what will happen to that. A part of me will always want to keep it, but I don't know how that will fit into my second life. I believe I will always keep the smaller urn I have but feel at a loss as to where it will be placed in the future. At some point I will have to go into the attic and figure out what to do with all the beautiful Christmas ornaments Denise kept. Many of them dated back to her childhood and some signified our time together.

I dreaded the thought that at some point everything that represented Denise would be set aside. Nonetheless, she will always have a place in my heart and someday, hopefully years from now, I will rejoin her both in heaven as well as here on Earth.

I have a moral obligation to carry on Denise's legacy. We will continue to hold our 5K race and have short and long-term goals for doing something Denise would be proud of.

I continue to change. I find myself becoming neurotic and seem to have a difficult time with short-term memory. Simple tasks like being able to walk away from a locked door prove challenging for me. I seem to struggle remembering to complete simple daily chores and fear that I will forgot something. I work to improve on this and hope I can continue to live without medication despite my personal struggles.

Finally, I feel deeply afraid of how having a second life will impact my connection to my first one. My life with Denise was so wonderful and I was so happy with where our lives were headed. As I continue to progress away from Denise, I struggle with guilt. I know moving forward will be hard, so I have to remind myself what Denise would have wanted for me.

I will always have internal issues with my part in this tragedy. I placed my trust in the doctors, enabling a bad situation to develop, and everything went horribly wrong. Afterward, they didn't have the decency to let me know they cared about me or my survival.

I hope this world always remembers Denise for how she lived rather than how she died. However, she would be relieved if this never happened again to another family. Someday God and I will discuss why He let Denise get to full-term with a new house, new car, and a smile that made this world better and then took her from us.

To Denise: I love you, I love you, I love you.

Acknowledgments:

I would like to thank all those people who reached out, got in a room with me, and provided much needed support. I will spend the rest of my life thanking you for all the support you gave me. I'm alive in large part because you were there for me.

I would like to give a special thank you to the following people: Mr. Bob, Teshia Utley-McKoy, Jeff Kent, Jared Boyer, Tim Morris, Dirk Wynne, Derek Hurdle, William and Anthony Lucas, Eileen Galligan, Lindsay Vollmin, Meredith Poole, Jeannie Simonds, Katie Ring, Mary Warren, Jennifer Lanane, Aileen Wala, Jessica Beisler, Ryan Blackwell, Thomas and Melissa Royer, Kevin Butler, the Gardinier family, the McKay family, the Huffman family, the Cawley family, and my amazing principal, Danielle Clark, who did such a great job helping me transition back into the classroom and the world.

Also, thank you to the people who greatly helped taking my words from the computer to this book: Jill Eagan, Drew Becker, and Diana Henderson.

I would like to extend my gratitude to all those people who gave me the gift of time. There are a number of people who just let me be. This book is to a large degree due to the fact that you gave me time to collect and organize my thoughts and to sit in front of the computer.

I would like to acknowledge the University of North Carolina Medical School for giving me a chance to talk about my experiences and for sharing my beliefs in the power of education. I know it wasn't easy letting me speak, but you all met, properly vetted me, and believed in me. I will always consider yours a world-class educational institution and medical school.

I would like to thank Denise for making me the man I am today. I sincerely hope I have made you proud.

About the Author

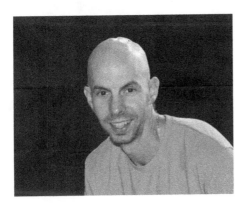

Levi Moore lives in Raleigh, North Carolina. He has his undergraduate degree and master's degree in Special Education. He has taught elementary Special Education for 14 years. Levi enjoys running, reading, and watching movies and sports. This is his first book. Levi is on Twitter @LeviMMoore.